HYSTERE

HYSTERECTOMY

A reassuring guide to surgery, recovery, and your choices

Jane Butterworth

Thorsons
An Imprint of HarperCollins*Publishers*

Thorsons
An Imprint of HarperCollins*Publishers*
77–85 Fulham Palace Road,
Hammersmith, London W6 8JB
1160 Battery Street,
San Francisco, California 94111–1213

Published by Thorsons 1995
1 3 5 7 9 10 8 6 4 2

© Jane Butterworth 1995

Jane Butterworth asserts the moral right to
be identified as the author of this work

A catalogue record for this book
is available from the British Library

ISBN 0 7225 3097 8

Printed in Great Britain by
HarperCollinsManufacturing Glasgow

All rights reserved. No part of this publication may be
reproduced, stored in a retrieval system, or transmitted,
in any form or by any means, electronic, mechanical,
photocopying, storage or otherwise, without the prior
permission of the publishers.

Contents

Introduction vii

1 Why is a Hysterectomy Performed? 1
2 Taking a Different Approach 27
3 Making the Decision 37
4 All About Hysterectomy 45
5 Getting Fit For Your Operation 56
6 In Hospital 69
7 Going Home 90
8 Hysterectomy, Hormones and HRT 101
9 Grief and Loss 114
10 Sex After Hysterectomy 121
11 A Last Word 128

Select Bibliography 130
Useful Addresses 133
Index 137

INTRODUCTION

A hysterectomy is the surgical removal of the uterus, or womb. After Caesarian section, it's the commonest women's operation, as, each year, around 70,000 hysterectomies are performed in the UK, and an estimated 1 in 5 of us will end up losing our wombs.

Different countries and different cultures have varying attitudes towards hysterectomy. During the 1980s, the proportion of women aged 50–54 who had had a hysterectomy ranged from 12 per cent in Sweden to 25 per cent in Australia and a staggering 33 per cent in the USA. The USA has consistently had the highest hysterectomy figures, although there is now a steadily growing band of medical opposition to the once-prevalent US view that hysterectomy is the first, rather than the last, line of medical defence.

The days when a hysterectomy was regarded as an enormous operation requiring a two-week stay in hospital are long gone. Advances in anaesthesia, hi-tech, state-of-the-art surgical equipment and keyhole surgery have meant that a woman having a hysterectomy in the 1990s often needs to remain in hospital for only a couple of days. The flipside of this is that sometimes hysterectomies are performed when they are not strictly necessary, or the answer to the problem.

We tend to regard doctors almost as gods, and in a way they are. On occasions they can literally hold our lives in their hands. Because of this we rarely question their opinions, and so if they suggest a hysterectomy as a way of dealing with a problem, we tend to accept their recommendation without demur.

There are occasions when hysterectomy *is* vital; it can be a life-saver or it can improve the quality of your life if your symptoms are unbearable. However, what it's sometimes easy to lose sight of is that, even with all the advances, it is still a major operation with all that involves, and it can have emotional after-effects, so the decision to have a hysterectomy shouldn't be taken lightly. The uterus is not just a useless organ like the appendix, even for a woman past child-bearing age. It is closely identified with being feminine and plays an integral part in our sexual and emotional health. Many women cannot lose such an important part of themselves without feeling some sense of loss and the need to mourn that loss.

A hysterectomy is not normally carried out to save your life unless the operation is for cancer, yet only 10 per cent of hysterectomies are performed for cancer. The majority of hysterectomies are performed for menstrual problems, many quite trivial, and although these problems may be uncomfortable and even painful, they won't kill you.

Although something may not be life-threatening, it can still be hell to live with, and a hysterectomy can seem like a tempting way out. There is no doubt that the commonest menstrual problem for which a hysterectomy is performed – heavy bleeding – can be debilitating in the extreme, and you may regard the loss of your womb as a small price to pay for being free of this problem. But, there are other treatments for this and it makes sense to be aware of these before you agree to a hysterectomy so you can make an informed choice.

This book looks at the problems that can lead to a hysterectomy

INTRODUCTION

being offered and the alternative treatments available. It examines the different types of hysterectomy operations that are performed, looks at the controversy surrounding the removal of ovaries and demystifies hospital procedures. Many women agree to have a hysterectomy without really knowing what it involves, or what the possible after-effects could be, because nobody has bothered to tell them. Sometimes these operations are desirable, sometimes essential, but often they're completely avoidable as many problems for which they are suggested can be successfully treated by means of medicines, alternative operations or natural or complementary medicine.

Doctors often suggest a hysterectomy because it's the easiest way round a problem that has so far resisted all previous attempts at orthodox treatment, and it has the added bonus of being a form of insurance against cancer of the reproductive organs, too. This is why many surgeons routinely take out a woman's cervix along with her womb, and many take out perfectly healthy ovaries as well, even in pre-menopausal women, simply because it's one less site for cancer. Whether this is necessary or justified is a matter for debate. Most women who have their healthy ovaries removed along with their wombs would never have gone on to develop ovarian cancer anyway, but I believe it should be the woman's choice – and only her choice – to have healthy parts of her body removed purely as a preventative measure against disease that might never strike.

Things are changing. Many doctors are no longer so ready to suggest a hysterectomy as a first resort and are much more open-minded about trying other forms of treatment. But, the better informed we, the patients, are the more able we are to press for other forms of treatment. Knowledge is power. The more you know, the more confidence you have when you need to make choices, and when you're faced with an important decision like whether or not to have a hysterectomy, you can make it secure in the knowledge that you're making the decision that is right for you.

Chapter 1
WHY IS A HYSTERECTOMY PERFORMED?

Although a hysterectomy is nothing like as dangerous as it was 30 years ago, it is still a major operation with all the attendant risks, including death. Even though some surgeons have started to use the minimum of invasive surgery, most do not, and many women who undergo it need a five- to seven-day stay in hospital and a recuperation period afterwards, which can be as long as three months, sometimes longer.

A hysterectomy is usually performed to treat relatively minor problems, such as menstrual disorders, the symptoms of which may be debilitating and distressing, but hardly life-threatening. It's a good idea to be fully aware of the problems for which a hysterectomy is normally recommended, because then you'll be in a better position to know whether or not there are other forms of treatment you can explore before you take the drastic option of surgery.

HYSTERECTOMY

Knowing Your Body

A woman's reproductive system consists of the uterus – a pear-shaped, expandable, muscular organ about 7.5 cm (3 in) long and 5 cm (2 in) wide – which is connected to her two ovaries by the Fallopian tubes. The cervix, or neck of the uterus, is situated at its lower end and joins the uterus to the top of the vagina, which opens to the outside.

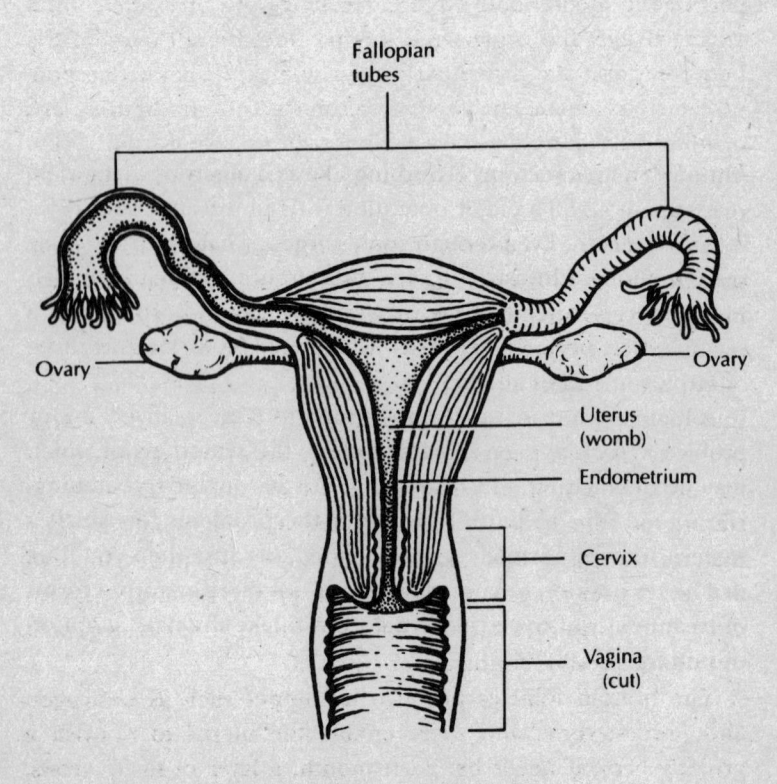

The female reproductive system.

WHY IS A HYSTERECTOMY PERFORMED?

When everything is functioning correctly, it's a triumph of design. The working of the system is governed by a number of chemical substances in the bloodstream called hormones, which act as our body's chemical messengers. Part of the brain – the hypothalamus – is responsible for controlling the output of these hormones, which are produced by the pituitary. The pituitary is a tiny gland situated at the base of the brain that automatically senses when hormones are needed and secretes them into the bloodstream accordingly. These hormones not only play a major part in the mental and physical workings of our bodies, influencing tissues and organs and linking up different parts of the body, they also play a vital part in our sexuality. They are responsible for our female characteristics, such as rounder figures, lack of body hair, and also the regulation of our menstrual cycles. Without them we would not be able to conceive and maintain a pregnancy.

The balance of hormones fluctuates throughout each menstrual cycle and it's essential that the balance is correct, as any imbalance can have a knock-on effect and produce a number of problems.

We are all normally born with our reproductive equipment intact, although dormant, including about half a million ovarian follicles – tiny sacs that contain all the eggs we'll need during our reproductive lives. Just before puberty starts, the hormone levels start to rise. The hypothalamus releases substances that stimulate the pituitary gland, and this causes the sex glands to develop and activate the sex organs. As a result, our ovaries develop and produce hormones of their own and start to release an egg each month for possible fertilization.

The ovarian follicles produce hormones such as oestrogen and progesterone, and these enable the uterus to nourish a growing baby, if needs be. Each month, a layer of tissue grows, thickens and becomes rich with millions of tiny blood vessels in preparation for pregnancy, under the influence of these hormones.

At the moment of ovulation, the developing egg breaks away from the ovarian follicle and is released into one of the Fallopian tubes, and if sperm is present it will fertilize the egg in the tube. The fertilized egg is then wafted along the tube towards the uterus, where it will attach itself to the uterine lining, which is called the endometrium. There it will grow, nourished by the thick, spongy endometrium that progesterone and oestrogen have prepared for a pregnancy. Progesterone also stimulates glands to secrete a nutritious fluid to nourish the egg.

If the egg is not fertilized, there is no pregnancy, so the levels of oestrogen and progesterone drop. Without these two hormones to support it, the endometrium shrinks and starts to disintegrate, and the muscular walls of the uterus start to push it and the unfertilized egg out through the uterus as a period. Then the whole cycle starts again.

Most of us will have around 400 periods between the menarche (the onset of menstruation in puberty) and the menopause, and so they are an important part of our lives. No longer are they universally regarded as a curse, surrounded by ill-founded and unpleasant myths, even though some women still believe wrongly that periods are in some way restricting. Nowadays more and more young girls and their mothers are seeing the onset of periods as a cause for celebration, the ushering in of womanhood.

A woman's reproductive system is a brilliant piece of natural engineering when everything's working without a hitch. Many of us, however, are not that lucky and if some malfunction tilts the balance of the hormones, menstrual disorders can occur. Most of the problems ultimately treated by a hysterectomy have their roots in a hormone imbalance of some sort.

What Can Go Wrong

Menstrual problems are very common. More than half of us suffer, or have suffered, from painful periods (dysmenorrhoea) or heavy bleeding (menorrhagia). A community survey of menstrual problems in Oxford discovered that half the 2500 women surveyed at random reported one or more menstrual problems, and 20 per cent had consulted their GP about these problems during the previous year.

It has been estimated that as many as 600 million working hours are lost each year because of painful periods, but heavy bleeding is the commonest symptom among women referred to gynaecologists. This is often a symptom of other underlying problems, but stress can also play a part. The menstrual cycle is governed by psychological factors as well as physical ones, and any upheaval in your life, such as divorce, bereavement of a loved one, moving house or losing a job, can have a physical effect.

Dysmenorrhoea (Painful Periods)

Most period pains feel like a dull ache in the lower abdomen or back, or manifest as cramps or contractions of the uterine muscle when the blood flow begins, but some women suffer from sickness, diarrhoea and such severe pain that they are unable to function properly for the first couple of days of their periods.

Primary dysmenorrhoea starts not long after the menarche – the start of the periods. The pain is caused by the strong muscles of the uterus contracting in response to increased amounts of the prostaglandins released to enable the unwanted endometrium to be expelled. This usually responds to painkillers and improves when a woman gets into her thirties. If it's really bad, your doctor can prescribe hormones or non-steroidal inflammatory drugs, like aspirin or ibuprofen, which suppress prostaglandins, or progestogen, such as Primolut N.

Secondary dysmenorrhoea is usually suffered by older women who've never suffered from painful periods in the past. This is a symptom of another underlying complaint, such as endometriosis or pelvic inflammatory disease (see pages 14–18). In this case, the pain is usually felt at the end of the cycle and gets worse as the next period approaches. It is constant rather than spasmodic and is usually felt deep in the pelvis rather than the lower abdomen. Your doctor will look for the underlying causes (see page 8) rather than treat the symptoms with painkillers.

What You Can Do

Strong painkillers like Nurofen can help. Exercises that involve stretching the muscles can help relieve spasmodic pain and contractions, and relaxation techniques, such as yoga, can have a beneficial effect. Some women have found that taking evening primrose oil, B-complex vitamins, or calcium and zinc supplements is useful, and homoeopathic remedies, including Aconite 30c, Chamomilla 6c, and Magnesium phosphate, which can be bought from chemists or healthfood shops, have also been known to alleviate pain. (See pages 33–4 for information on homoeopathy.)

Menorrhagia (Heavy Bleeding)

Menorrhagia is usually caused by fibroids, but it can also be caused by endometriosis, pelvic inflammatory disease, polyps, IUDs (intrauterine devices, such as the coil) or a hormonal imbalance. If the bleeding occurs between periods or after the menopause, it *must* be investigated as it may be a sign of endometrial cancer, although this is a relatively rare form of cancer (see pages 22–23).

Very often, however, it happens because our perfectly balanced hormonal systems start to break down. As we approach the menopause, the rhythmical cycle begins to go awry and our ovaries may sometimes fail to release an egg each month. If there is no ovulation, there is no progesterone, which means that the endometrium cannot be shed as normal. As a result, the oestrogen-producing follicle disintegrates and, as it does so, the oestrogen level falls and the endometrium is shed. But it is not shed in response to the drop in progesterone, as happens in the normal menstrual cycle, but because of the lack of oestrogen. This makes the bleeding irregular, heavy and prolonged.

The amount of blood lost during your period varies, although however much you lose it's normally the same each month. The usual blood loss is about 60 ml (over 80 ml and it's considered heavy). Most of us haven't a clue how much blood we lose, but a good yardstick is that if normal sanitary protection can't cope with the flow, it's time to see your doctor. You should also always see your doctor if there is a sudden increase in the amount of blood you're losing, as this might mean there's an underlying medical cause.

Studies that have measured menstrual loss have shown that some women believe they are losing far more blood than they actually are, and a large proportion of the women attending gynaecological clinics complaining of heavy bleeding were not suffering from clinically defined menorrhagia, that is, more than 80 ml blood loss. Nevertheless, many went on to have a hysterectomy.

Anyone who has ever suffered from really heavy bleeding will know the misery it can cause, and how washed out it can make you feel. At its worst, it can lead to anaemia. I once bled so heavily I could only go out wearing four night-time towels, and even those had to be changed after an hour. On one occasion, I dared not set foot outside the house, I was so worried about leaking. Every time I got up from a chair, I surreptitiously inspected the seat to see whether or not I'd left a stain. I felt uncomfortable, wiped out and depressed, so much so that if my doctor had suggested a hysterectomy during that time I'd probably have agreed gratefully without a moment's thought, just to put an end to such wretchedness. Fortunately, he didn't and the problem righted itself with a combination of progestogen treatment, evening primrose oil and homoeopathic remedies, but the experience gave me an insight into why hysterectomy can seem very appealing at times.

If your periods suddenly become heavy and you are not heading towards the menopause, this could indicate an infection, fibroids or a hormonal imbalance, but many women have very heavy periods with no abnormal physical cause. One woman I spoke to had had extremely heavy periods since the age of 11, and maintained that the happiest day of her life was when she had a hysterectomy at the age of 42 and realized she would no longer have to go through such monthly menstrual misery.

Diagnosis and Treatment

If the blood loss has increased suddenly, doctors will want to find out what is causing it. You may be asked to measure your blood loss. This can be useful because, as we saw, a lot of women overestimate the amount of blood they lose simply because it looks a lot when it's soaked into a pad, so, once the actual loss has been measured and they are reassured that the amount is absolutely normal, they no longer regard it as a problem.

Doctors will usually carry out a pelvic examination for any disorder relating to the reproductive system. This is not the most pleasant of experiences, but it's not painful or even uncomfortable as long as you're relaxed. You lie on your back with your knees bent and apart, and the doctor will place a small instrument called a speculum into your vagina to hold open the vaginal walls. He or she will then insert two gloved fingers of one hand into your vagina while pressing down on your abdomen with the other. This enables the examining doctor to feel for any ovarian cysts or abnormal growths in the uterus.

WHY IS A HYSTERECTOMY PERFORMED?

A dilation and curettage (D & C) is a minor operation performed under general anaesthetic. It is often recommended as a way of investigating heavy bleeding. It involves stretching the neck of the uterus and scraping out some of the lining with a spoon-shaped instrument called a curette. Samples, or curettings, are sent for analysis, and this is useful for diagnostic purposes because the curettings can be tested for cancer of the endometrium. It's also a way of diagnosing fibroids. Removing part of the endometrium can also sometimes solve the problem and alleviate the bleeding, at least in the short term.

New Techniques

Some doctors now suggest an endometrial biopsy instead of D & C because it can be done under a local anaesthetic. This involves endometrial tissue samples being taken using an instrument that is passed through the cervix into the uterus.

A hysteroscope – a lighted viewing instrument that is inserted through the cervix – is starting to be used to diagnose endometrial or uterine problems as it enables the doctor to get a clear view of the uterine cavity.

Endometrial resection is another fairly new way of treating heavy bleeding, which involves the removal of some or all of the endometrium with a resectoscope. This is a slender telescopic instrument with a small heated wire electrocautery loop on one end (see pages 42–3).

Other Treatments

Sometimes certain tablets can alleviate bleeding problems, although some can cause worse symptoms than those they are prescribed to alleviate, so be sure you fully understand the potential side-effects. The combined contraceptive pill can be effective, as can progestogens such as Primolut N (norethisterone) and Duphaston (dydrogesterone), but progestogens can have side-effects for some women, such as weight gain, bloating, breast tenderness and breakthrough bleeding. Danazol, a synthetic hormone, works well at decreasing blood loss, but it has so many unpleasant side-effects, such as masculinization, voice deepening, weight gain, decreased breast size, facial hair growth and depression, that many women prefer not to take it. Some of these side-effects are irreversible. There are also drugs that stop the body from making prostaglandins, such as Ponstan (mefanamic acid), which is taken during menstruation.

If you're approaching the menopause, it might be that your hormones are starting to malfunction as the system starts to shut down, and a follicle stimulating hormone (FSH) blood test can confirm this. FSH is produced by the pituitary gland to ripen the ovarian follicles during a normal menstrual cycle. As you head towards the menopause, FSH levels usually rise because the ovaries are less responsive to FSH, so more is produced to encourage them to work. If you are nearing the menopause, therefore, the problem should eventually cure itself.

Fibroids

Fibroids are frequently the root cause of heavy bleeding, and the commonest reason for a hysterectomy being performed. They are solid growths of muscle and fibrous tissue that grow on the uterus, and it's estimated that 20 per cent of all women over 30 have them – indeed, some research has suggested that the figure may be as high as 40 per cent. Many don't even know they've got them until a doctor feels them during a pelvic examination, as they often cause no problems and virtually never become cancerous. So, don't let the threat of cancer scare you into having surgery for fibroids if they are giving you no problems.

Fibroids grow inside the wall of the uterus (intramural fibroids), outside the wall (subserous fibroids) or inside the lining of the uterus (submucous fibroids). Intramural fibroids are usually trouble free, unless they grow large and start taking up

WHY IS A HYSTERECTOMY PERFORMED?

more than their fair share of room. Submucous fibroids can cause heavy and painful periods. Subserous fibroids can be painful if they grow large enough to press against other organs, especially during menstruation, and sometimes a fibroid can grow out on a stalk, which can become twisted and cause a lot of pain. Fibroids can cause infertility if there are a lot of them and they grow large, and that's when they need to be removed.

Fibroids grow when they're stimulated by oestrogen, so they shrink and eventually disappear after the menopause, unless the woman is taking hormone replacement therapy. The early contraceptive pills, which contained high doses of oestrogen, have been linked with fibroid growth, but today's low-dosage pills shouldn't cause such problems.

Although most fibroids don't cause symptoms unless they grow large – about as big as a five-month pregnancy – if they do grow that large, they can cause severe pelvic pain or pressure on the bladder and bowels, and very heavy periods.

Drugs that suppress ovarian function and reduce oestrogen levels can shrink fibroids. These are known as luteinizing hormone-releasing hormone (LHRH) agonists. LHRH is a chemical produced by the hypothalamus that influences the ovaries' production of oestrogen, and LHRH agonists are synthetic versions of these hormones, which can shrink oestrogen-related tumours such as fibroids. These can often stop periods altogether, though, and so should not be taken for a long time without hormone replacement therapy, as they can cause menopausal symptoms.

Other Forms of Surgery

Surgery is usually the only real answer for large and troublesome fibroids, but there is an alternative to hysterectomy. This is an operation called myomectomy, during which the surgeon removes the fibroids through a cut in the uterus. This is virtually a routine operation in France, yet it is often difficult to find a surgeon to perform it in the UK and the United States.

This is because it is a difficult operation with a higher complication rate than hysterectomy, and a lot of surgeons haven't been trained to perform it. It requires a great deal of skill as in less than skilled hands it can lead to internal scarring. It takes a great deal longer than a hysterectomy, and is a more dangerous operation because there's a slight risk of uncontrollable bleeding during the operation, because each fibroid has to be carefully separated from the uterus and detached from its blood supply.

Furthermore, it may only provide a temporary solution, as sometimes fibroids can grow again after a myomectomy, particularly if surgeons leave behind the smaller fibroids, which they sometimes do to prevent scarring. Small wonder, then, that so many surgeons prefer the cheaper, safer alternative of a hysterectomy, but it is worth trying to find one that can at least offer you the choice.

Some gynaecologists perform myomectomies with the aid of a laparoscope, which is a thin telescopic-like surgical instrument inserted through a tiny incision near the navel. The fibroids can then either be vaporized by laser or cut into pieces and removed, and this removes the problem of uncontrollable bleeding as a laser seals rather than scars.

Because lasers can go deeper into tissue than can a surgeon, the fibroids can be totally removed, including their seedlings, and they won't recur. However, this is a long and costly operation requiring a very skilled surgeon to perform it and, at the time of writing, it is not yet widely available in the UK.

A new and less invasive form of treatment enables small fibroids to be taken out through the vagina. A hysteroscope (a lighted viewing device inserted into the uterus through the cervix) can be used along with a laser or a wire loop to cut or shave off small fibroids from the uterine wall.

It is important to remember despite these various options, however, that many fibroids cause no problems at all, and yet some doctors still try to persuade women to have a hysterectomy

WHY IS A HYSTERECTOMY PERFORMED?

because of them. They claim that large fibroids make it difficult to feel ovarian tumours during pelvic examinations and so there is a risk of missing ovarian cancer, a rare but often deadly disease. But ovarian tumours can be detected using ultrasound or CAT scans if malignancy is suspected. Unless fibroids are causing you trouble, there is absolutely no need to have them removed.

What You Can Do

The growth of fibroids is stimulated by oestrogen, and the amount of oestrogen in a woman's body can be influenced by the amount of fat in her diet. Women whose diet contains high levels of fat have, on average, a third more oestrogen in their blood than women on low-fat diets. Thus, fibroids are rare in underdeveloped countries where the diet consists mainly of high-fibre grains and vegetables. Obesity also increases a woman's oestrogen levels, as body fat converts women's male hormones into oestrogen.

Eating a low-fat diet made up largely of vegetables, fruits and starches can help. Californian doctor John McDougall maintains that changing to such a diet can cause oestrogen levels to fall by more than 30 per cent in a few weeks, and reports that in his own practice in California he has observed symptoms of pain and excessive bleeding disappear in a matter of weeks after putting his patients on such a diet. A low-fat diet will also help you lose weight, and so reduce oestrogen levels even more.

Supplements of bioflavinoids with vitamin C can strengthen blood vessels, and many women have reported a significant reduction in flow after taking them for only three months, but little is known about the long-term effect of these supplements. Natural sources are safest and the ones richest in bioflavinoids are citrus fruits, grapes, apricots, tomatoes, broccoli, peppers, cherries and rosehips.

Endometriosis

Endometriosis is the most common gynaecological disorder after fibroids and is a major cause of infertility and painful periods, yet little is known about this distressing condition. It's caused when the endometrium – the lining of the uterus – starts to grow on other parts of the body, usually on the outsides of the ovaries, uterus and Fallopian tubes, but sometimes the bowel, bladder, and even the lungs, ears and eyes, may be affected, too. If the tissue is found *inside* the muscle of the uterus wall, this is known as adenomyosis.

Endometriosis can affect any woman of child-bearing age, and there can be as many as a hundred patches of endometrial tissue or as few as one. This tissue can't become cancerous, but normally it causes excruciating pain because the patches of tissue respond to the hormones produced each month during the menstrual cycle, growing, thickening and shedding blood.

Unlike the normal monthly period during which the endometrium is shed, this blood has nowhere to go. Because it can't escape, it can cause inflammation and pain, blood-filled ovarian cysts or a build-up of scar tissue, which can cause the nearby organs, such as the uterus or bowel, to stick together. The most usual symptoms of endometriosis include painful periods, other pelvic pain, painful sex and painful ovulation, depending on where in the body the patches are growing. It's a chronic, progressive condition that can result in infertility.

Diagnosis and Treatment

Endometriosis can be hard to diagnose as the symptoms are similar to those of other diseases and it can't be seen on an ultrasound scan.

It's usually diagnosed by means of a minor operation called a laparoscopy, which is carried out under a general anaesthetic. While you're asleep, carbon dioxide gas is pumped into your abdomen through a small incision by your navel. This separates your pelvic organs so they can be seen more easily. The surgeon then inserts a laparoscope – a slender, lighted, telescope-like instrument, into your abdomen, which shows up the growing tissue patches and the extent of the scar tissue. If the endometriosis is mild it can be treated at the same time by cauterizing it, although this is a highly skilled procedure as it is necessary to avoid damaging the organs on which the tissue is growing.

Surgery

Severe endometriosis can be treated during a laparotomy. This is a major operation during which the abdomen is opened by making an incision just below the bikini line, in a similiar way to a hysterectomy. Sometimes women are asked before being given a laparoscopy for their consent in case a laparotomy is needed, to save going through another anaesthetic if the laparoscopy diagnoses such severe endometriosis that it can only be treated by means of a laparotomy.

Laser surgery can be used to remove large patches of endometriosis, and this works well because it burns off the tissue deposits without damaging the organs on which it is growing. A laser-equipped laparoscope, which has been pioneered by Dr Camran Nezhat at the Northside Hospital, Atlanta, Georgia, is an exciting development in the treatment of endometriosis. Because the laparoscope only needs a tiny incision to be made (so the abdomen is not opened up) and lasers seal off the blood vessels, there is less risk of infection, scarring, bleeding and pain. However, this requires the surgeon to be highly skilled and the operation is not yet widely available.

Medicines

Progestogens such as Primolut N or Duphaston, which stop ovulation and menstruation, are often used because these trick the body into thinking it's pregnant, and with no oestrogen to nourish them, the tissue patches shrink.

Danazol (danol) is a hormone that reduces the oestrogen levels in the body by inhibiting the production of hormones by the pituitary gland, bringing about a temporary false menopause. It's very effective, but the drug itself can have severe side-effects, including masculinization. Also, some of these side-effects are irreversible, even after you stop taking the danazol. Gestrinone (dimetriose) is similar to danazol.

A hysterectomy is usually suggested when medicines and all else fails, but it won't solve the problem if there are tissue deposits on other organs, unless the ovaries are removed as well. Even that doesn't always work, because if only a tiny piece of the ovary remains, it will generate oestrogen. Hormone replacement therapy (HRT), which is usually given after a total hysterectomy and oophorectomy, can occasionally reactivate previous sites of endometriosis.

What You Can Do

Taking vitamin supplements can help – especially B-complex and B6 – to combat the side-effects of hormone treatment. Evening primrose oil can relieve pelvic pain and heal scar tissue. Zinc promotes healing and fertility, and selenium ACE relieves pain and other symptoms and enhances the immune system.

Vivienne relates her experience:

I've suffered from heavy and painful periods since I was a teenager, but it got so unbearable after I had my second child I went to see my doctor. He diagnosed endometriosis and tried me on progestogen, but that didn't work at all, and I didn't want to try danazol because I'd heard it had a lot of side-effects. He sent me to see a gynaecologist, and when I told him nothing had worked he said, 'You'll just have to have a hysterectomy then'. There was no discussion, he didn't even ask me what I thought. I absolutely freaked out and said no way, not without trying other things. So I got in touch with the Endometriosis Society and they sent me a list of alternative treatments to try and I started on evening primrose oil, various vitamin pills and a natural supplement. After about four months, I started to see some improvement. I won't say it's cured, but it's a lot better and I can put up with it – particularly as at 47 I'm nearing the menopause, and when that happens there won't be a problem any longer.

Pelvic Inflammatory Disease

Pelvic inflammatory disease (PID) is a collective term for inflammation or infections of the Fallopian tubes, ovaries, cervix or uterus. It often starts in the tubes and can be caused by an IUD, pelvic surgery, sexually transmitted diseases like chlamydia or, occasionally, after an abortion if an infection develops.

There are four types of PID:

- *acute* PID – a severe infection with symptoms that include a high temperature and severe abdominal pain
- *sub-acute* PID – a less severe form of acute with milder symptoms
- *chronic* PID – which both acute and sub-acute can become if they're left untreated, which can go on for years and result in a general feeling of ill health, which never seems to clear up
- *recurrent* PID – where attacks are interspersed with periods of feeling well.

If it isn't treated, it can travel all through the reproductive system and lead to infertility, usually due to the scar tissue or adhesions it can cause on the Fallopian tubes. Not only do sufferers have a poor quality of life, PID can lead to peritonitis if left untreated – and this can be life-threatening.

Diagnosis and Treatment

Because symptoms can be similar to those of other diseases, PID can be hard to diagnose. In order for it to be properly treated, the organism causing the infection needs to be identified by taking a vaginal swab and then treated with antibiotics. Sometimes even antibiotics can't always cure chronic PID, and a hysterectomy may be suggested if this is the case. Partial surgery is sometimes considered before hysterectomy – that is, the removal of the diseased or scarred organ.

What You Can Do

If you get intermittent attacks, keeping yourself in good health can help, as can avoiding stress and getting enough sleep. Some women have found that cutting out alcohol, cigarettes and coffee is helpful, together with taking vitamin supplements.

Prolapse

Prolapse is the term used to describe the falling or sagging of an organ, usually the uterus. The pelvic organs, which include the bladder, uterus and bowel, are supported by a sort of sling of muscles, ligaments and other tissues that stretch from the pubic bone to the bottom of the spine. As the uterus grows during pregnancy, the strain on the supporting ligaments and muscles can be so great that, after childbirth, these muscles don't always return to their former taut state. Because of this, the pelvic organs aren't held in place as well as they should be and they start to sag. Prolapse can also occur in women who are severely overweight or after the menopause when tissues and muscles start to lose their tone and may start to weaken.

If a prolapse is very severe, the uterus can drop straight through the vagina or can descend at an angle and press forwards on the bladder or backwards on the bowels and rectum. The vagina can also prolapse independently of the uterus.

WHY IS A HYSTERECTOMY PERFORMED?

Symptoms include:

- a dragging sensation or heaviness in the back or lower abdomen
- a feeling of looseness in the pelvis
- incontinence
- frequent desire to urinate even though the bladder is empty
- difficulties with penetration during intercourse
- constipation.

Treatment

A ring-shaped pessary that fits into the vagina to hold the uterus in place can work well, and many older women prefer this to surgery, even though it needs to be changed every six months. Often a prolapse causes no problems at all and is best left alone, but if it does start to cause problems, a repair operation – which involves lifting the weak tissue to improve muscle tone – can be performed, to give better support.

Many of those with a severe prolapse are beyond child-bearing age, and so a hysterectomy rather than a repair operation is more likely to be suggested. However, it is not always a good idea because it doesn't repair the weak and sagging ligaments that cause the problem, and many women suffer a further prolapse after their hysterectomy. To get round this problem, some surgeons tighten up the ligaments, but then they can be so tight that sex is painful.

What You Can Do

If the prolapse is mild, you can improve your pelvic muscle tone by doing pelvic floor exercises (see pages 62–3), although nothing will help a complete prolapse other than surgery. Losing weight, taking regular exercise and eating a diet high in fibre can also help. HRT may be prescribed if the problem is caused by lack of hormones after the menopause.

Cancer of the Reproductive Organs

The only time a hysterectomy is absolutely essential is when cancer has been diagnosed.

Cervical Cancer

Cancer of the cervix, or neck of the uterus, is completely curable if caught in its early stages. It is the only cancer that can be prevented, as smear tests can pick up cell changes or abnormalities on the cervix long before cancer develops.

Unlike other cancers of the reproductive organs, cervical cancer has a clearly defined pre-cancerous stage, which is called cervical intraepithelial neoplasia (CIN). This indicates that there are changes in the cervical cells, and these changes are normally graded according to severity, as follows.

- CIN 1, which means that there are only very minor cell changes. These sometimes disappear spontaneously, but you should have another smear test in three to six months to make sure.
- CIN 2, which means that there are moderate cell changes. This should always be treated immediately (see under Diagnosis and Treatment below).
- CIN 3, which means that there are severe cell changes, but they are still not pre-cancerous.

Micro-invasive cancer means that cancer is present, but only in the cervix and it can sometimes be treated by having a cone biopsy (see page 21). Invasive cancer is actual cervical cancer and it is for this (and usually micro-invasive cancer as well) that a hysterectomy is recommended. If it is undetected, it can spread to the vagina and neighbouring tissue, and right through the pelvis – then a hysterectomy is inevitable.

It is thought that cervical cancer is linked to sexual activity, as

WHY IS A HYSTERECTOMY PERFORMED?

it is virtually unknown among nuns. Those who had their first intercourse at an early age and have had a lot of sexual partners are at higher than normal risk. Other risk factors are smoking, herpes, genital warts, and having an uncircumcized partner. It doesn't mean you'll get cervical cancer if you have nodded your head to all these factors, but you do have a slightly higher than average risk and so it's wise to have regular smear tests.

Symptoms
Bleeding after sex and in between periods or after the menopause is the commonest symptom. There may also be a discharge.

Diagnosis and Treatment
Pre-cancerous conditions can be treated with laser or cryosurgery (where the affected tissue is frozen). If the disease is more extensive, a cone biopsy may be performed, which involves removing a cone-shaped section of tissue from the centre of the cervix to check how deeply the cells have spread into the cervix. If the cancer cells *have* spread, even if they are only confined to the surface tissue of the cervix and are not invasive, a total hysterectomy will be recommended. If the cells have spread to below the surface of the cervix and cancer has developed, a radical, or Wertheim's, hysterectomy is a must. This involves removing the top half of the vagina, cervix, the ligaments that support the uterus, lymph glands and some tissue, as well as the uterus, Fallopian tubes and, usually, ovaries.

Joan recalls:

I had laser treatment after a positive smear test, and then received a letter telling me the cells had not yet been removed. The doctor wrote, 'I cannot tell you that you haven't got micro-invasive cancer'. They can only go so far with a laser, you see. I can't describe how I felt, other than terrified. I'd only ever been into hospital to have my tonsils out when I was a child, and I've always been very nervous of anything like that. But cancer . . . then I read on: 'It is clear you need a total abdominal hysterectomy'. I told the doctor, who was a delightful man, that I didn't think such a letter should have been sent. It's too stressful; that sort of news should be told you face to face, you need to talk about it and to discuss the options. It upset me so much because we'd never talked about this possibility, he'd always skirted round it. I think I assumed that as I'm a naturally healthy person it would go away on its own. A friend, who is a natural health practitioner, was up in arms. She said don't do it, try alternative therapies. I might have put it off if it had been CIN 1, but not with the possibility of it being invasive cancer.

Endometrial Cancer

Cancer of the endometrium usually only occurs in post-menopausal women, and the strongest risk factors are obesity and a high-fat diet. Doctors believe it could be linked to high oestrogen levels as women who took HRT in its early days, when it consisted solely of oestrogen without progestogen, have been found to be at a higher risk of endometrial cancer.

Pre-cancerous changes in endometrial cells should always be checked out as the abnormal proliferation of these cells can lead to cancer. In most cases, pre-cancerous lesions wouldn't progress to cancer even if left untreated, but they must always be treated, just in case.

Symptoms
The most important symptom is abnormal bleeding, especially after the menopause. Any alterations to a woman's normal menstrual pattern or post-menopausal bleeding should be investigated.

Diagnosis and Treatment
Tissue samples from the endometrium need to be tested, and so a D & C is usually performed under general anaesthetic. This is

WHY IS A HYSTERECTOMY PERFORMED?

a minor operation that involves scraping out some of the endometrium with a spoon-shaped instrument called a curette, and sending the tissue for analysis (see page 9).

Some doctors use an endometrial biopsy instead of a D & C because then tissue samples can be taken under a local anaesthetic (see page 9). Smear tests do *not* pick up endometrial cancer.

Ovarian Cancer

Cancer of the ovaries is less common than cervical or uterine cancer, yet it causes more deaths than either and is the fifth leading cause of death from cancer in women.

It causes a lot of anxiety to doctors and women alike, because it has few symptoms until it is so far advanced it is virtually untreatable. The disease can be detected in its early stages by ultrasound and routine pelvic examinations, but most newly diagnosed cases are in advanced stages and so the five-year survival rate is less than 20 per cent. Because of this, a lot of doctors routinely remove ovaries during a hysterectomy, especially in women over 40 (see page 53), as this removes a potential cancer site.

The development of ovarian cancer has been linked to the use of talcum powder or menstrual debris, and women who have had no children are thought to be at slightly higher risk. It is predominately a disease of older, post-menopausal women, with 90 per cent of the cases occurring after the age of 45, and although there are no conclusive heredity factors, there seems to be a family link. If your mother or sister had ovarian cancer, you have a higher than average chance of developing it yourself. Diet seems to play a part, too. The rate of ovarian cancer among Asian women, which is a lot lower than their American or European counterparts, rises to the same level among those who emigrate to the West.

HYSTERECTOMY

Symptoms
As we have seen, most women have no symptoms if the cancer is in its early stages, other than perhaps some vague pelvic discomfort or abdominal pain or swelling. Often the tumour is discovered during a routine pelvic examination.

Diagnosis
If your doctor feels a mass in your abdomen during an examination, you'll probably be sent for an ultrasound scan, which can show up a tumour or cyst. A skilled doctor can generally tell whether or not it's a benign tumour or a cyst at this stage, but, if there is any doubt, you may be sent for a computerized axial tomography (CAT) scan, which is a sort of X-ray that can confirm the diagnosis and show the size and position of the cancer. A chest X-ray, blood tests and analysis of any lung or abdominal fluid that might have accumulated can also be carried out. A laparoscopic biopsy may also be performed (see pages 14–15 for a description of a laparoscopy), during which a small tissue sample is taken for analysis.

Treatment
There are four main stages in the development of ovarian cancer:

1) growth limited to one or both ovaries
2) growth spreads from the ovaries to the pelvis
3) the cancer extends to the rest of the abdominal organs, but not the liver; most women with ovarian cancer are diagnosed at this stage
4) the cancer has spread to the liver and other sites.

The cancer is also graded according to its aggressiveness. Slow-growing tumours are graded as 1, whereas fast-growing tumours, which spread quickly, are graded as 3. Treatment is determined

WHY IS A HYSTERECTOMY PERFORMED?

by both grade and stage.

Surgery for stage 1 ovarian cancer is effective, but usually both ovaries are removed along with the uterus and Fallopian tubes, even if only one ovary is affected. No chemotherapy is usually given for stage 1 cancer, but it's essential that you consult a surgeon who is an expert on ovarian cancer. Radiotherapy can be used after surgery, if any tumour remains.

When the disease is in its later stages, chemotherapy is the main treatment after surgery has removed as much of the growth as possible.

An anticancer drug treatment called Taxol™ was launched in 1994 and this has given hope to women with advanced ovarian cancer. It works by stopping the cancer cells dividing and growing, by promoting the assembly and stabilization of what are called microtubules within cancer cells. By encouraging the proliferation of these microtubules, Taxol™ prevents their breakdown and the cell dies as a result. Clinical studies have consistently demonstrated that Taxol™ can exert an antitumour effect in those patients whose cancer has failed to respond to other therapies, so the picture is not as bleak as it once was.

Hormone Replacement Therapy
If your ovaries are removed, you will immediately go into a surgically induced menopause, the symptoms of which will be much more dramatic than is the case when menopause occurs naturally, which it does over a number of years. HRT is an effective way of treating menopausal symptoms, but it is essential that it is prescribed by a specialist (see pages 107–13). You can help alleviate symptoms by taking evening primrose oil supplements and maintaining a good diet.

When is a Hysterectomy Necessary?

The conditions described above are those for which a hysterectomy is usually recommended. Cancer is normally the only disease for which it is *essential*, although there are other complaints that can so damage the quality of your life as to make a hysterectomy seem like the only answer. You won't die of heavy periods, for example, but, certainly, they can make you feel so ghastly you'd settle for virtually anything to relieve them.

The majority of hysterectomies are performed to relieve symptoms that are *not* life-threatening. Most are not for chronic disease or disease that cannot be treated any other way. So, it's worth seeing if any of the alternative treatments can help your problem or alleviate your symptoms before you take such an irrevocable step.

Chapter 2
TAKING A DIFFERENT APPROACH

Ask almost any alternative medicine practitioner how they're doing and the chances are they'll say they're doing very nicely, thank you. For the truth is that more and more of us are shunning orthodox medicine, which often may not have the answer to our particular problem, and turning to natural or alternative medicine. Orthodox medicines, the side-effects of which can be worse than the complaint they have been prescribed for, the soaring cost of prescriptions and the rise in stress-related and psychological illnesses, for which orthodox medicine, more often than not, has no answer, have all helped to popularize alternative medicine.

Complementary medicine is, by and large, safe and non-addictive, whereas various new drugs have been brought out over the years that manufacturers claim have been thoroughly tested yet have gone on to cause terrible side-effects. And who knows what the long-term effects of many drugs will be?

Many of us have come to see broad-spectrum antibiotics as a cure-all and feel deprived if our doctor won't give us a prescription for them, even for something as mild as a sore throat. We try to suppress colds or flu by taking painkillers or anti-inflammatory drugs rather than letting the disease take its course, because we don't want to put up with the irritating symptoms. When the symptoms have gone, we think we're better, but, often, we're not – we've just bought ourselves a bit more time before the next virus or infection comes along because we haven't got to the root of the problem.

Even the mildest medicines can have side-effects: aspirin can irritate the stomach lining, prolonged use of paracetamol can cause liver damage; penicillin can cause life-threatening allergies; antihistamines can make you drowsy; some antifungal drugs can occasionally impair your liver function; some tranquillizers are addictive; hormones can masculinize you; antibiotics can kill your 'friendly' bacteria as well as unfriendly invading bacteria, and so impair your immune system. No such risks exist with natural remedies, as long as they are prescribed by qualified practitioners and taken properly, as most of them have been in existence for thousands of years.

Of course, there are occasions when orthodox medicines *are* necessary, even life saving, and antibiotics *do* work. Anybody who's seen the almost miraculous way antibiotics can clear up infection in a matter of days can't blame people for seeing them as a cure-all. And complementary medicines won't save you if you've got a ruptured appendix or need a hysterectomy for cancer – although it's arguable that if you do all you can to lead a healthy life by eating a highly nutritious diet, avoiding pollutants and managing your stress, your chances of ever needing surgery should diminish.

The holistic approach to medicine involves looking at the *whole* person, not just the part that's ill or the symptoms. This is because the theory behind holistic medicine is that we are whole beings – body, mind, spirit and emotions. Inside us is a vital force, or energy flow, that affects the way we feel. If we are in good health, that energy flow is perfectly balanced and so we feel content, full of vitality and strength. If we become ill, the balance is

TAKING A DIFFERENT APPROACH

disturbed and the symptoms of sickness are produced. Most menstrual problems have their roots in a hormone imbalance, and how well our hormone system works is related to our state of mind – stress can play havoc with it. Stress can suppress ovulation and raise the level of oestrogen, and that, in turn, can stimulate the growth of fibroids with their accompanying symptoms.

The treatment of symptoms alone may make you feel better for a while, but if you don't find the root cause of them they're likely to return. For example, if you have heavy bleeding, your doctor may well prescribe progestogen. This is likely to reduce the blood loss, but the *cause* of it remains – and the likelihood is that the symptom will be back, just as soon as you stop taking the progestogen. The aim of holistic medicine is to cure the whole patient, not just get rid of the symptoms.

Holistic practitioners don't just suggest a natural remedy you can take. They work on the principle that everyone is different and so are their needs, and so the first consultation will probably consist of a long and detailed interview in which you'll be asked not only about your medical history, but your whole way of life, and a whole lot of other things you may feel are unrelated. A holistic practitioner tries to build up a picture of you as a complete person, and your state of mind is important, too, because when we do become sick or our bodies malfunction, we must play an important part in the healing process.

There are many different forms of complementary medicine and some natural medicines *can* be used for symptomatic relief from menstrual problems, but practitioners try to understand you as a person and prescribe for you on that basis, as well as trying to discover the cause of any imbalances. You can't be impatient with complementary medicine, because it takes time to work. Furthermore, natural medicine is only part of a healthy way of life. There is little point in hoping it will make you better if you carry on insulting your body by having a stressful lifestyle, eating junk food, taking no exercise and smoking and drinking. No amount of natural medicine will keep you in good health unless you look at your whole lifestyle.

Complementary medicine works best if it is able to work *alongside* orthodox medicine, and many doctors are becoming much more open-minded about therapies they might once have dismissed as quackery. Some doctors are also homoeopaths and, if the occasion arises, they treat certain things with natural homoeopathic remedies rather than orthodox medicines. The British royal family must take some of the credit for helping homoeopathy to become recognized as having a part to play as they have long been enthusiasts of it: the Queen is Patron of the Royal London Homoeopathic Hospital and her family has been using this form of medicine for generations.

Natural medicine can never replace orthodox medicine, however, and, to give credit where it's due, advances in orthodox medicine have played a large part in prolonging our life expectancy. Deaths occurring during childbirth, for example, held back female life expectancy until the 1930s, when the discovery of antibiotics, safer anaesthetics and blood transfusions all combined to significantly lower the mortality rate. Equally, it would be a foolhardy person who attempted to treat cancer with only natural medicine. But, orthodox medicines and surgery should be treated with caution and respect, and used only when absolutely necessary, not as a panacea for every twinge and ache. It is sometimes all too easy when you've got depressing menstrual problems to see a hysterectomy as a way out and it's tempting to go along with the doctor's verdict. Be patient for a little longer. Unless you've been diagnosed as suffering from cancer, if no form of orthodox medicine has worked, it's worth trying a natural alternative. It might save you from having a hysterectomy – and avoiding major surgery where possible has to be a good thing.

TAKING A DIFFERENT APPROACH

Acupuncture

Western medicine is based on the principle of attacking the invading bacteria with medicines such as antibiotics, but, in so doing, it also suppresses the body's own immune function: in effect, it fights against the disease *and* the body.

The Chinese way of healing is to regulate the system and *boost* the immune function so the body can withstand invading germs and weaken their attack. Then, after the attack has subsided, the body does not have to muster all its immune functions to fight against the disease.

Chinese medicine sees the body as a balance between two opposing but complementary natural energies – yin and yang. Yin is associated with passivity, cold, darkness, inwardness and rest; yang is associated with excitement, heat, light, activity. Any imbalance of the two is believed to cause illness and disease, and acupuncture aims to correct this disharmony by using needles to stimulate specific points on the body. These 300 or so acupuncture points lie along invisible energy channels, known as meridians, which are rather like stations on a railway line. Each has an association with a particular body part. Acupuncture needles are used to try to increase or decrease the flow of energy or life force – known as *ch'i* – through the meridians.

A practitioner arrives at a diagnosis after taking a careful history of your condition, including your emotional as well as your physical state – indeed, every facet of your life, although menstrual problems are less influenced by outside forces than others. Although some of these questions may seem irrelevant, all have a purpose. Your pulses will be felt at both wrists and your tongue carefully examined, as it is a useful indicator of your general health. When the acupuncturist has decided where the disharmony in your *ch'i* lies, needles will be inserted into various points. It's usually quick and painless, although you might feel some

HYSTERECTOMY

sensation for a short while.

Susan, an acupuncturist, talks about her work:

Most of my patients come when they've been to the doctor already, and they've usually tried drug therapy and it hasn't worked. They're the ones who feel instinctively that because there isn't anything terribly wrong with them, drastic solutions seem to be inappropriate. If you're told you've got cancer, you accept that surgery is appropriate. If you're having heavy bleeding, it isn't. It looks to me like a sledgehammer to crack a nut. Acupuncture can help because it can stimulate your natural hormone production.

If you allow the body the opportunity to correct itself, unless the situation is very severe, it will do a jolly good job getting itself back on course. It's a bit like a new car – if it splutters and grinds to a halt, you take it to a garage to be fixed, you don't say take the engine out.

With Chinese medicine, you're trying to estimate the condition of health that exists in the person, unlike a Western doctor who says this disease looks like this, that disease looks like that. I'm not describing fibroids in Chinese words, I'm describing what the patient might be experiencing which could be explained in Western terms by her having fibroids. Basically, she'd report symptoms of very heavy flow and a lot of pain, and I'd try and diagnose what has led to this, and there may be a combination of causes. I wouldn't treat the symptoms of fibroids, I'd encourage the ch'i *to flow well and effectively and then her own body, which has incredible restorative powers, will do it for her.*

I've had patients come in and tell me they've been diagnosed by their GP as having fibroids, and I treat them and the symptoms get better. Now, I don't know if their fibroids have shrunk, all I know is they're better because they're not bleeding as much as they did.

The worst of it is patients come in and say, 'Oh, I feel much better, but I've been to see the doctor and he says I've still got fibroids, and I've got to have them out even though they're not presenting a problem'. I prefer to take the standard model body complete with all its bits and that's what I'd like to end up with. What human being can say a uterus or an ovary is unnecessary and we can live without it?

The majority of acupuncturists are lay practitioners (that is, they are not medically qualified) and, in theory, anyone can set up as an acupuncturist even if they have had no recognized training. It is important, therefore, to ensure that you choose an acupuncturist who belongs to one of the professional bodies affiliated to the Council for Acupuncture (see page 134), as these organizations have high standards of training and a strict code of practice. Some medical doctors go on to train in acupuncture, and you can get lists of these doctors from the British Medical Acupuncture Society (see page 133).

Homoeopathy

Homoeopathy is based on the principle of treating like with like. It was popularized by German doctor Samuel Hahnemann at the beginning of the last century when he noticed that a herbal remedy for malaria produced malaria-like symptoms when taken by a healthy person. He concluded from this that the symptoms of illness were the body's attempts at fighting infection, that medicines which *produced* the same symptoms of illness could help *recovery*, and that drugs which *suppress* symptoms only *deny* the body the chance to cure itself.

As with acupuncture, the aim is for the body to stimulate its own powers of healing. This can take some time, so you can often feel worse before you feel better. The remedies are derived mainly from plants and minerals, and they are safe and non-addictive. Dosage is vital, and the lower or more highly diluted the dose, the more potent the remedy. Although you can buy ready-made remedies over the counter in chemists or healthfood shops, the most effective remedies are only available from qualified homoeopaths, who base their prescriptions not only on a careful medical history, but also on your lifestyle, personality, and physical and emotional make-up.

As with acupuncture, there are lay practitioners and qualified medical doctors who have gone on to train in homoeopathic medicine. Homoeopathy is more closely aligned with orthodox medicine than any other form of natural medicine, a significant number of GPs work within the NHS and there are five NHS homoeopathic hospitals. To find a medically qualified homoeopath, contact The Faculty of Homoeopathy (see page 136). To find a lay homoeopath, write to The British Homoeopathic Association for a list, enclosing a stamped, self-addressed envelope (see page 136).

Ann tells her story:

I'd suffered from severe period pain for 20 years. It was so bad I was virtually bed-ridden for a day a month and I tried everything – naturopathy, yoga, acupuncture, diet, you name it. Then I moved and my new GP was homoeopathically qualified, so he tried me on a variety of homoeopathic remedies. I took these for a year or so and, although there wasn't much improvement for at least six months, it did ease it quite significantly in the end.

A couple of years later, it became bad again and I had a lot on. I couldn't spare the time homoeopathic treatment needs so, reluctantly, I agreed to take Primolut N. Even more reluctantly, I have to admit that this worked almost miraculously, as it stopped the problem almost overnight. But homoeopathy did work for a while, and I often regret not sticking with it.

TAKING A DIFFERENT APPROACH

Herbalism

The healing power of herbs has been known for thousands of years and modern medicine owes a lot to herbalism: many modern drugs are derived from herbal remedies. Although herbalism can be used symptomatically, as with other forms of natural medicine, it is most effective when it is used holistically, that is, prescribed by a herbalist who is treating the whole person rather than just the disease and who is endeavouring to discover the root cause of the symptoms and then restore the balance of your health.

Remedies are often mixtures of several herbs, and they can be potent. Some can be dangerous, even though they are derived from natural sources. You shouldn't take herbal remedies for longer than a couple of weeks without supervision, especially if you can see no improvement in your condition. To find a herbalist, send a stamped, self-addressed envelope to the National Institute of Medical Herbalists (see page 135).

A Final Note

There are many other forms of natural or alternative medicine, but acupuncture and herbal-based medicine are probably the most effective in the treatment of menstrual problems. Don't expect any form of natural medicine to work immediately, and note that often the symptoms can worsen before they get better. If one sort of natural medicine doesn't work it's worth trying another, as what works for one person sometimes doesn't work for you. Also, sometimes a combination of two or more therapies can be the answer.

Natural remedies cannot harm you, providing they are prescribed or administered by qualified practitioners. And they may

HYSTERECTOMY

end up alleviating your symptoms so much that surgery becomes unnecessary. That possibility alone should make them worth considering.

Chapter 3
MAKING THE DECISION

Whether or not you choose to have a hysterectomy and what sort you have is influenced by a number of factors:

- the reason it's been recommended
- the symptoms you've been having
- your tolerance level as far as your symptoms are concerned
- your personality, attitudes and expectations
- whether or not your GP decides to refer you to a surgeon, rather than try to treat the problems that have occurred with drugs or other therapies
- the surgeon's attitude towards hysterectomy – whether they see it as a first or last resort form of treatment
- whether or not your local hospital is equipped with hi-tech, state-of-the-art diagnostic equipment, so the exact nature and extent of the problem can be clearly revealed and there can be no mistaken diagnoses.

Rita relates her experience:

HYSTERECTOMY

I had my hysterectomy 30 years ago when there was no sophisticated equipment to diagnose what was wrong. I was 34 and had suffered from heavy periods. The doctor diagnosed a large fibroid and said a hysterectomy was the only way. Even though I didn't want any more children, it was a shock, but I accepted what he said as gospel. You did in those days – doctors knew everything, or so we thought. Even when I'd had the hysterectomy and it was discovered there were no fibroids, I felt no resentment. At least it stopped the problem.

Some gynaecologists see the uterus as a pointless part of a woman's anatomy once she's finished her family, and suggest a hysterectomy as a first rather than a last resort because it removes a potential cancer site. It's easy to go along with this, but the fact is that it's *not* just another organ. Although being feminine is not dependent on having a womb, it can play an important part in our sexual responses (see Chapter 10) and some women do feel the loss acutely. Think about whether or not your symptoms are so unbearable that a hysterectomy is the only way to free yourself from chronic and debilitating problems.

Caroline had the following experience:

I'd been having problems since I was sterilized. I bled constantly, took all sorts of drugs which didn't work, and the specialist said it was problems with my ovaries and it sometimes happened after a sterilization. He said I could be suffering like this for 20 years before I started the menopause, because I was only 32 at the time. Either that or I could have a hysterectomy. I chose a hysterectomy, and they actually found the problem was with my womb, which was double its size.

It wasn't a hard decision – my mother and sister were in their thirties when they had theirs, so I thought I can put up with this. I was lucky because I had it done by a surgeon who had just perfected a new, non-invasive technique, but I would still have had it done whatever technique they'd used, even though my sister had been so ill after she'd had hers. I knew what to expect. Afterwards I felt fantastic and was back at work within three weeks, entirely due to this technique. I have never regretted it at all. It's made such a difference to my life; I can't describe to you the misery of constant bleeding. It's fantastic.

But not all women survive this operation so well, and it can have a deep and far-reaching impact. All major operations can leave you feeling vulnerable and depressed, but hysterectomy is different because many women see the womb as the essence of their femininity. One study of women who had undergone a hysterectomy revealed that they saw menstruation and its identification with youth, femininity and sexuality as a significant loss once it had gone.

Sarah tells her story:

I had no choice but to have a hysterectomy because I was diagnosed as having invasive cancer of the cervix. The shock of taking that on board was bad enough, but that was almost nothing compared to what followed the actual operation. I went through a very long and painful time when I felt as though part of my femaleness had gone and I wasn't a complete woman, even though my rational self told me this wasn't so and thousands of women have this op. I became clinically depressed, although some of it was to do with the cancer, and it took many months of counselling and support before I could see my way out of that dark period.

Give Yourself Time

It's sometimes difficult to think straight when a hysterectomy is suggested. It's often a totally unexpected shock and it takes a while for it to sink in, which is why it's a good idea to take your partner or a friend along to the consultation. It can be a while after the appointment that questions you wish you'd asked start forming in your mind. If you are referred to a specialist for any persistent menstrual disorder, be prepared for them to suggest a hysterectomy and make a list of any questions you want answered before you agree to it. Examples of questions to ask the doctor are the following.

- Why has a hysterectomy been recommended?
- Are there any suitable surgical alternatives?
- Have I been told about all the non-surgical treatments available?
- What sort of hysterectomy do you propose doing?
- Do you perform this technique regularly?
- Will my ovaries be left in place? If not, why not?
- Will my cervix be removed?
- Will my vagina be shortened?
- What could go wrong?
- What after-effects might I suffer?
- How long can I expect to be in hospital and how long will I be convalescing?
- When can I go back to work?

Questions to ask yourself include the following.

- Have I already finished my family or might I want a baby some time in the future?
- Are my symptoms so unbearable a hysterectomy is the only option?
- Have I tried all the alternative treatments available?

MAKING THE DECISION

You and Your Partner

Don't rush into making any sort of decision until you've talked it through with your partner. Not only will his support make you feel more secure and less isolated, it will give him an opportunity to voice any fears and anxieties *he* might have. Some men are alarmed at the idea of a hysterectomy, which involves the removal of an organ they see as so closely linked to the femininity of their partner. They need information and reassurance.

It'll also give the two of you the chance to talk about any ideas you might have about having further children. Some couples don't realize until a hysterectomy is recommended that they'd like to have a baby.

If you've been suffering from really bad problems, you may be quite relieved at the thought of a hysterectomy, especially if you've explored every other possible form of treatment. But, before you make the decision, ask your surgeon about new and less invasive surgical techniques that are starting to replace the traditional hysterectomy operations.

New Surgical Alternatives

These new techniques involve taking away the endometrium but leaving the uterus intact – known as endometrial ablation. The destruction of the endometrium has been tried using chemical methods, but these have now been abandoned because of their unreliability and toxicity. The focus now is on hysteroscopic surgery, during which the surgeon removes the endometrium using a laser or by means of electrocautery, aided by a telescopic instrument called a hysteroscope, which is inserted through the cervix.

The trouble is that these techniques need to be performed by a very skilled surgeon, and there have been reports of inexperienced surgeons putting patients at risk by performing these techniques without sufficient training. One woman suffered serious damage to her urinary system after a resectoscope (the instrument used to cut away her endometrium) perforated her uterus. The good news, though, is that doctors are currently starting a £4 million keyhole surgery retraining programme, and some predict that by the end of the 1990s three-quarters of all operations will use the minimum invasive techniques necessary – saving thousands of women from major operations. The real bonus of these techniques is that they can often be performed under local anaesthetic, the patient can be back at home within a matter of hours, and back at work within days. Unfortunately, at the time of writing, they are only available at certain hospitals.

Transcervical Resection of the Endometrium (TCRA)

TCRA, or endometrial resection, is one of the most popular new techniques. After the surgeon has inspected the uterus with a hysteroscope and deemed it suitable for this technique (it's no good if you have large fibroids), an instrument called a resectoscope is passed through the cervix into the uterine cavity. This is similar to a hysteroscope but it has a heated wire loop at the end that shaves away the endometrium and any fibroids as well, and both doctor and patient can watch the proceedings on a monitor because there's a tiny camera on the tip of the instrument.

You can either have a partial resection, which results in lighter periods as part of the endometrium grows back, or a total resection, which involves the complete removal of the endometrium, after which your periods will stop completely. The whole process takes about 20 minutes.

In a study done on 24,354 women who had been suffering excessive and painful bleeding and were treated with this method, 90 per cent reported pain-free lighter menstrual cycles. TCRA doesn't always eradicate period pain, but it does seem to alleviate it in varying degrees.

Endometrial Laser Ablation

This is the permanent destruction of the top layer of the endometrium by laser, but the healthy tissue underneath is not damaged in the process. A hysteroscope is inserted through the cervix into the uterus together with a laser, and the surgeon works using a monitor linked to a miniature video camera. It's similar to a D & C, but more effective because more of the lining is removed, and because the laser seals off blood vessels as they are cut so there is little risk of blood loss. It can also be performed under a local anaesthetic.

Sometimes the patient is given danazol four to six weeks before the operation to shrink the endometrium, as this makes treatment easier and more effective. Periods may return after this treatment, but, if they do, they are likely to be much lighter and less painful – but the woman will be left infertile.

Critics of this method say that it fails to deal with the disease behind the symptoms and so is only really useful for certain conditions, such as small fibroids. More worryingly, some maintain it can mask diseases.

Radio Frequency-induced Endometrial Ablation

This is similar to laser ablation except that the endometrium is destroyed using low-frequency waves, such as those generated in microwave ovens. A probe is inserted into the uterus by the surgeon and this is then attached to an energy source. It burns away the endometrium with radio frequency energy.

HYSTERECTOMY

The Pros and Cons

If they are used for certain conditions, such as heavy bleeding or small fibroids, these techniques seem to work well, with patient satisfaction being as high as 100 per cent in many cases following the operation. Although temporary feelings of pain and discomfort can follow, as is normal after any operation involving the uterus, these are usually shortlived.

Even if these techniques are performed under general anaesthetic, because they involve no abdominal incision and only last between 15 and 30 minutes, the quantity of anaesthetic administered is minimal and so recovery time is quicker. Some, as we have seen, can be carried out under a local anaesthetic. Time spent in hospital can range from a matter of hours to a couple of days, and convalescence is usually between one and two weeks. You can be back at work within a fortnight.

However, although many surgeons had hoped that these new techniques would partially replace traditional hysterectomy, the long-term results are poor in a third of cases. The technique may need to be repeated within five years, although that's something most women would be prepared to put up with. Your periods may return, and although bleeding can be reduced or often eradicated, you may still be left with painful periods.

Although you may not be rendered infertile after such treatments, some studies show a higher than average risk of miscarriage.

The long-term effects of these techniques are yet to be seen, but most experts believe that they are an important breakthrough in the treatment of heavy bleeding – and the most important advantage of these techniques is that they treat the problem but leave your uterus intact.

Chapter 4
ALL ABOUT HYSTERECTOMY

Once, an abdominal hysterectomy, which involves the removal of the organs through an incision in the abdomen, was performed more or less routinely, with the occasional vaginal hysterectomy being carried out for a prolapse. Nowadays, there are a lot more options available.

The successful introduction of the laparoscope – a thin telescopic instrument that allows the surgeon to view the abdominal cavity and also provides an image on a monitor – has allowed surgeons to devise a new way of performing a hysterectomy using this remarkable piece of equipment. Even though 80 per cent of all hysterectomy operations are still performed in the traditional way, laparoscopically assisted hysterectomy is becoming more widely used.

Now a hysterectomy can be performed:

- through an incision in the abdomen
- through the vagina
- through the vagina, but with the assistance of a laparoscope inserted through the abdomen for part of the surgery
- through the vagina, using a laparoscope for all the surgery.

HYSTERECTOMY

What Sort?

What sort of hysterectomy you have is determined by the reason for your having it, your age, and your surgeon's preferences and skills. Be sure to ask your surgeon exactly what the operation suggested involves, what techniques will be used and why that particular operation is being recommended. When you sign the consent form, be sure it specifies exactly what will and will not be removed during the operation. Some surgeons remove ovaries routinely, for example, even in pre-menopausal women, which is something you should only consent to after a great deal of discussion and having been given information on the possible after-effects of such an operation (see page 53).

The various kinds of hysterectomy are as follows:

- *sub-total hysterectomy* when the uterus is removed but the cervix, ovaries and Fallopian tubes are left in place, but most surgeons prefer not to perform this type of hysterectomy because the cervix is a potential site for cancer, so, if you have this operation, you must carry on having smear tests afterwards
- *total hysterectomy* the commonest operation, when the uterus and cervix are removed but the ovaries and Fallopian tubes are left
- *total hysterectomy with bilateral salpingo-oophorectomy* when the uterus, cervix, ovaries and Fallopian tubes are removed, which many surgeons favour for post-menopausal women, even if their ovaries are perfectly healthy, as an insurance against ovarian cancer
- *radical, or Wertheim's, hysterectomy* when the uterus, ovaries and Fallopian tubes are removed, as well as the upper part of the vagina, the ligaments that support the uterus, the lymph glands and some fatty tissue, which is normally only

ALL ABOUT HYSTERECTOMY

1. Total hysterectomy (most commonly performed)

The whole of the womb and the cervix are removed and the ovaries are left behind.

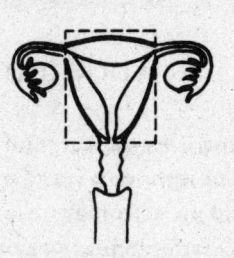

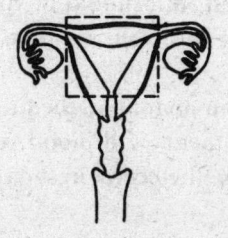

2. Subtotal hysterectomy (rarely performed nowadays)

The main body of the womb is removed but the cervix and ovaries are left behind.

3. Total hysterectomy with bilateral salpingo-oophorectomy

The womb, cervix, both ovaries and fallopian tubes are removed.

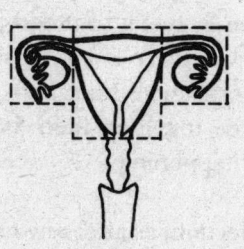

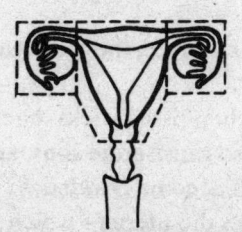

4. Radical (Wertheim's) hysterectomy

Same as in 3. together with removal of the top of the vagina, surrounding fatty tissue and glands (lymph nodes).

The various kinds of hysterectomy.

performed when invasive cancer is present.

Let us now look at each of these types of hysterectomy in more detail.

Abdominal Hysterectomy

This involves the surgeon making an incision in your abdomen. If it's to remove a very large fibroid or other abdominal mass, a vertical incision may have to be made. Otherwise, most surgeons use a Pfaffenheim horizontal incision, which is below the bikini line. The small, neat scar you will be left with should be hidden by your pubic hair. It's worth checking with your surgeon what sort of incision will be made.

Once the surgeon has opened up your abdomen, the uterus is then cut away from its supporting ligaments and blood vessels, and the vagina is carefully cut away from the cervix in such a way that its length should not be affected.

This is such a common operation that complications are rare. However, there is some risk attached to all operations requiring a general anaesthetic and, as women's pelvic organs are situated so close together, there is a chance of the following complications happening:

- infection, as after any major operation
- injury to the bowel or bladder
- injury to the urethra, the tube that connects the kidney to the bladder
- adhesions, or scar tissue, which is when tissue sticks together after surgery (endometriosis can also cause adhesions, and these can cause the pelvic organs to become bonded together – for example, the bowel to the uterus – which can make it difficult for the surgeon to separate them)
- post-operative bleeding.

Vaginal Hysterectomy

Performing a vaginal hysterectomy without the aid of a laparoscope is usually only done when a woman has a prolapse, and then a great deal of skill is required as the potential for doing damage is immense.

With a vaginal hysterectomy, the surgeon cuts away the uterus from its supporting ligaments through the vagina, and then pulls it out whole or else cuts it up and takes it out in pieces.

A vaginal hysterectomy has fewer complications than an abdominal one, the hospital stay is much shorter – two to four days on average – and, because there is no abdominal incision, recovery is a lot faster.

If the technique is performed by a skilled surgeon, complications are rare, but the following can happen:

- infection
- bladder and bowel injuries
- adhesions – if there are bad adhesions as a result of previous abdominal surgery or pelvic inflammatory disease (see pages 17–18), the surgeon may well not try to perform the operation vaginally and open up the abdomen.

Laparoscopically Assisted and Total Laparoscopic Vaginal Hysterectomy

This is an alternative to an abdominal hysterectomy, not vaginal hysterectomy. A laparoscope is inserted through a tiny abdominal incision in the navel, enabling the surgeon to get a good view of the abdominal cavity. The hysterectomy is then performed using the laparoscope to cut the uterine ligaments, and the uterus is either removed intact or dissected and then removed through the vagina, and the cervix is then sewn up in the traditional way.

This sort of hysterectomy has advantages in that it avoids major abdominal surgery and so needs shorter hospitalization and recuperation time, although the operation can take much longer than a traditional abdominal hysterectomy. Because the surgeon has such a clear picture of what's going on, any bleeding or blood clots can be spotted. Adhesions and endometriosis can be excised and ovaries removed using this technique. A laparoscopic hysterectomy may be considered for stage 1 endometrial, ovarian and cervical cancer.

Apart from the faster recovery time, the advantages of having your hysterectomy performed in this way include a reduced risk of infection and a virtually non-existent risk of intestinal obstruction, which can occasionally happen after major abdominal surgery. However, it is more difficult and more time-consuming than a vaginal or abdominal hysterectomy and, unless it is performed by a proficient surgeon, can have a high complication rate: in one study it was as high as 60 per cent.

In 1992, surgeons at Graduate Hospital, Philadelphia, Pennsylvania performed the first total laparoscopic hysterectomy in the USA. As with a laparoscopically assisted hysterectomy, the laparoscope is inserted through the navel, providing an image of the abdomen on a monitor. Two tiny incisions are then made on either side of the pelvis and, through these, the instruments to detach the uterus, Fallopian tubes and ovaries, if necessary, are inserted. When these organs have been detached, they are removed through the vagina.

A laparoscopic hysterectomy can take up to three hours' operating time, which is more than three times longer than a traditional vaginal or abdominal hysterectomy, but patient recovery time is far shorter and there is less risk of trauma to nearby tissue because of the clear image the surgeon has. According to Dr Harry Reich, who pioneered this technique, about 90 per cent of all hysterectomy operations could be performed laparoscopically.

The Future

Consultant Gynaecologist Cheng Lee has perfected an even less invasive hysterectomy technique at Rochford Hospital, Canvey Island, Essex. He performs all his hysterectomy operations vaginally, without even the assistance of a laparoscope.

Mr Lee's technique is a modified version of that first performed by Irving Rayner in 1988 in Houston, Texas. He has developed a form of surgery that he uses for most conditions requiring a hysterectomy, apart from cancer. He removes the uterus and ovaries vaginally using his experience as a surgeon rather than a laparoscope to guide him. He says about his technique:

> *I don't believe laparoscopic hysterectomy is that good because it can have complications. All operations have a complications rate, but whereas it is 4–6 per cent with abdominal hysterectomies, with our technique it is only 2 per cent. The really revolutionary thing about this is that the woman is out of hospital and home within 24 hours of having the operation, compared to the traditional hospital stay of 7 days.*
>
> *I've modified some of the steps, which may seem simple but are very important – techniques in controlling bleeding, so you don't need a pack or catheter.*

He has also minimized the after-effects of anaesthesia on his patients, which must be an important factor in his patients' astonishingly rapid recovery, as it's anaesthesia which can cause the most profound and far-reaching after-effects. He uses an epidural (spinal) anaesthetic as well as a general anaesthetic, which means his patients need lighter general anaesthesia.

HYSTERECTOMY

Mr Lee continues:

I get a lot of opposition. There's no such thing as a free lunch, and this operation takes one hour or one hour ten minutes compared to the half an hour a traditional abdominal hysterectomy can take, so that means more theatre time and more anaesthetic is needed. In the UK, we're conservative and slow to change. We're behind regarding HRT; in the USA they're 30 years ahead of us.

All Mr Lee's patients I spoke to referred to him in almost reverential tones. All had been discharged from hospital the day after their operation with none of the weakness or side-effects often reported after a normal hysterectomy. One even drove herself home after her hysterectomy, which is almost unbelievable. But, at the time of writing, Mr Lee is the only surgeon practising this technique in the UK, and as this is a very skilled and specialist procedure, there is great potential for complications if it's performed by a less skilful surgeon.

Caroline tells of her experience of Mr Lee's technique:

I arrived at the hospital on Monday morning at 8 o'clock. The operation was performed at one, and when I woke up I felt fine. Later on that afternoon, when I was back in the ward, I asked for the drip to be taken off. That night I got up and went to the loo and had a fag – I felt wonderful! The next day I was up, dressed, bathed and waiting for Mr Lee's visit. When he came, he told me to lift up a chair, which I did, and then to walk over to the end of the ward and back to him. He took me down the corridor and told me to run up and down stairs, and it was incredible, I could.

Twenty-four hours after I'd had my operation, my sister collected me. When I got home I made dinner, hoovered and did the ironing and, far from feeling ill, I didn't feel as though I'd had anything done to me. I thought my stomach would be tender but it wasn't. It was as if I'd been to the dentist. At work, nobody believed

I'd had a hysterectomy!
From day one I didn't stop doing anything. I could have driven myself home, and I went back to work a week later. My work involves computing, filing, some lifting, and a lot of shift work. I could pick my son up, carry anything. I don't regret it, it's sheer bliss.

What's Right For You?

Most surgeons have their own preferences as to how they perform a hysterectomy, and it's not a good idea to try and persuade one who rarely performs a vaginal hysterectomy to do so. If a less than experienced surgeon attempts a vaginal hysterectomy, there is a risk that other organs might be damaged. If you are particularly keen on having a vaginal hysterectomy and your surgeon is not a specialist in the particular techniques required to do one, you'd be best finding another surgeon who does specialize in them.

The Ovarian Controversy

Some surgeons routinely remove ovaries during a hysterectomy, even when they are operating on pre-menopausal women with perfectly healthy ovaries. They argue that there is little point in leaving a potential cancer site when it no longer serves any useful purpose. In the USA, 45 per cent of women have their ovaries removed during a hysterectomy, whatever their age, and yet it is not usually necessary to remove the ovaries of a menstruating woman during a hysterectomy. Removal of the ovaries, or oophorectomy, can have far-reaching effects: unless the woman is given expert HRT afterwards, she will undergo an immediate surgical menopause.

It's true that ovarian cancer is one of the most insidious and deadly cancers, because it shows few obvious symptoms until it has spread so much it cannot be successfully treated. However, it is usually only found in post-menopausal women and is relatively uncommon. Studies have shown that over 7000 oophorectomies need to be performed to prevent 1 death from ovarian cancer, so the possibility of having the disease is fairly remote.

Many women are frightened into accepting their surgeon's advice and agree to their ovaries being removed, but it's a decision that shouldn't be taken without being fully aware of the consequences. The symptoms of a surgical menopause are far more severe than those of a natural menopause, which happens over an extended period of time, and the younger the woman, the worse the symptoms.

Doctors will argue that HRT can make up for this, and routinely put in hormone implants during the operation (see Chapter 8). But, ovaries are highly intricate organs with many functions that can never be entirely replaced by HRT, and the success of HRT itself lies in the skill of the dispensing doctor and many doctors know little about this complicated subject.

Even if a woman is past the menopause, the ovaries still go on producing small amounts of hormones, including testosterone, all of which are responsible for sexual desire and overall feelings of well-being. Although the adrenal glands carry on producing testosterone, it's not enough to make up for that which has been lost from the ovaries.

Doctors remove the cervix during hysterectomy for similar reasons. However, with regular smear tests giving early warning of pre-cancerous changes, is this really necessary? Recent research suggests that taking away the cervix can interfere with a woman's sexual enjoyment as the cervix has been identified as a source of sexual pleasure, and some doctors are starting to rethink this whole area and to leave the cervix in place when performing a hysterectomy.

Having healthy ovaries and a normal cervix removed as a precaution against cancer that may never develop should be a decision that the woman concerned should take, after weighing up the arguments for and against, not the doctor alone.

How to Choose

In an ideal world, we would be able to make an informed choice as to exactly what sort of operation we should have in consultation with the surgeon. Unfortunately, it's not that simple. Many of us don't ask for more information before surgery and many doctors don't talk to their patients beforehand about what their options are. What sort of hysterectomy you end up having depends on:

- the reason you're having it
- the skill and preferences of your surgeon
- your overall state of health
- the willingness of your GP to refer you for a second opinion
- how assertive and well informed you are.

Don't be dictated to. Ask questions, gather as much information as you can. Find out exactly why your surgeon has suggested one particular sort of operation rather than another and if you are unhappy about the option recommended and feel strongly about having another type, ask to be referred to another surgeon for a second opinion. This is such an important decision it's not one that should be taken hastily or without a great deal of research and thought.

Chapter 5

GETTING FIT FOR YOUR OPERATION

Unless a hysterectomy is being performed for cancer, the majority of women have to wait weeks or months before they are given a date for their operation. This time can be put to good use by getting yourself in good shape, mentally and physically. The healthier you are when you have the operation, the quicker you'll heal and be back to normal, and the less likely you are to suffer side-effects and complications.

If you're significantly overweight, diet. The heavier you are, the more anaesthetic you'll need and the longer it will take to recover. Also, too much fat makes the operation technically more difficult and makes it difficult to get your stomach muscles strong again afterwards. It's important, too, that you're mentally healthy and have accepted that the operation is something you really want, that having it is the right decision for you. If you go into hospital with anything other than a positive frame of mind, you're likely to come out depressed and your recovery time will be longer.

The Importance of Diet

Our state of health is influenced primarily by our lifestyle. Smoking, pollution, bad diet, drinking excessive amounts of alcohol, stress and lack of exercise can all take their toll on our health.

Most of us don't eat enough fresh vegetables, fruit and grains – rich sources of carbohydrates, fibre, calcium, vitamins and minerals. One-fifth of men in Scotland eat no fruit at all. Yet, a low intake of vegetables and fruit not only means we miss out on vital nutrients, many studies have shown that the nutrients in fruit and vegetables have a protective effect and can lower our risk of disease.

A good diet should be the norm for everyone, but it's all the more important in the run up to your operation. Avoid processed foods, convenience foods and foods that are high in fat, salt and sugar. Eat fish, chicken, whole grains and plenty of fruit, vegetables and beans. Instead of using fat to cook and dress food, use olive oil as it is an unsaturated fat with positive health benefits. Virgin olive oil contains a substance called oleic acid and this, taken daily, can protect the body from harmful organisms, such as fungal infections. Garlic is a wonderful natural antiseptic that promotes healing, is good for the digestion and, if you make it part of your daily diet, can help protect against infection.

The antioxidant vitamins C, E and beta-carotene, which are found in fruit and vegetables such as citrus fruits, rosehips, tomatoes, blackcurrants, green peppers, cauliflower, broccoli and sprouts, play a major part in mopping up destructive free radicals. Free radicals are byproducts of natural metabolic processes and are normally kept under control by our body's natural antioxidants, so there is no problem. But, free radicals also occur as a result of outside sources – poor diet, lifestyle and some medical conditions – and if they increase to such an extent that our antioxidant levels cannot neutralize them, the excess free radicals attack the body's cells and cause tissue damage. Free radical damage has been linked to the development of a wide range of chronic, degenerative disorders.

As we age, more free radicals are produced, our defence system weakens, cell damage builds up and produces age-related changes, and the risk of infection and diseases rises. It makes sense, then, to build up your body's immune system by eating highly nutritious food so your body is in peak condition before surgery.

Yogurt has been renowned as a health-giving food for thousands of years, because of the protective effect is has on our intestines. Our normal intestinal flora consists of groups of micro-organisms, including lactic bacteria, or lactobacilli. These are very important as they transform sugar into lactic acid, creating a favourable environment that arrests the development of toxic bacteria, including candida, and protects the intestinal mucus against the invasion and activities of harmful micro-organisms. Lactic bacteria are also able to produce certain B-complex vitamins.

In old age, bad or putrefactive microflora start to accumulate in the intestines due to the reduced secretions of the digestive glands and this can lead to an increased production of toxic bacteria. Products of lactic acid fermentation such as yogurt restore the 'friendly' intestinal flora, which can stop the 'unfriendly' flora from proliferating and restore the correct balance. Yogurt is easy to digest and contains more protein and riboflavin than milk. Make sure it's unsweetened and made from skimmed milk, however, or it can be high in calories.

Smoking

The last time I was in hospital, I got talking to a woman who was in for what was a relatively minor operation for most people, but was hazardous for her because she smoked an unbelievable 100 cigarettes a day. This had resulted in such a diminution of her lung capacity that she had only about one-third of her lung function remaining. As she was telling me all this, half an hour before they were due to take her down to theatre for her operation, she was smoking a cigarette. I could hardly believe it.

I didn't see her again because she was taken to the intensive care unit (a move almost unheard of after such an operation, but her breathing difficulties had made anaesthesia very dangerous in her case), so I'll never know if she survived. But I do know that by continuing to smoke at such a level, she had put her life in danger to the extent that minor surgery had become, in her case, life-threatening.

The drawbacks of smoking are so well documented as to be common knowledge – smokers know that every cigarette shortens their life by five minutes, to say nothing of constricting the coronary arteries, raising the blood pressure, damaging the bloodstream's oxygen-carrying capacity and impairing the immune system. They're probably sick of people handing out advice telling them to stop smoking. But, if you really, really won't give up, for your operation's sake stop for a couple of weeks before you're due to go to hospital. If you don't, you'll be at greater risk of a chest infection, you're likely to have more problems with the anaesthetic, you're at greater risk of developing complications such as blood clots or chest infections after your hysterectomy, and you'll almost certainly take longer to recover. The plain fact is that smokers are unhealthier than non-smokers.

Exercise

If your hysterectomy involves any sort of abdominal incision, the stronger your stomach muscles are before the operation, the easier it will be to get back into shape again afterwards than if the muscles are slack and the flesh flabby. Check with your doctor first that it's OK to exercise.

Once you've got the all clear, each day do the following exercises.

Stomach Exercises

The following two exercises are difficult and you may not be able to manage them at first, but it's worth persevering. Try the gentle crunches to start with if you prefer. Do as many sit ups and crunches or gentle crunches as you can each day before your operation, and you will develop stomach muscles strong enough to withstand the rigours of surgery without being ruined for life. You'll also get closer to that seemingly unobtainable ideal of a flat stomach.

Sit Ups

Do as many as you feel able to, but don't overdo it. Try to increase the number each day. Don't do this exercise if you have any sort of back trouble or just after a meal. The exercise builds up the upper stomach muscles.

- Lie on the floor with your feet hooked under a bed or held down by an accommodating partner or friend.
- Put your hands behind your head with your elbows out to the sides, keep your knees slightly bent to avoid straining your lower back, then slowly sit up, using your stomach muscles to raise your upper body from the floor. Try to touch your

knees with your nose.
- Hold the position for a moment, then slowly lie down again.

Crunches

This is a difficult exercise, but keep trying as the results are worth the effort. Repeat as often as you can, aiming to increase the number you can do each day.

- Lie down on the floor with your legs bent at the knees and your feet crossed at the ankles. Your knees should be facing towards the ceiling.
- Link your hands behind your head to support your neck, then lift your head and shoulders off the floor as much as you can, using your stomach muscles to lift you rather than your arms and looking up at the ceiling.
- Lift as high as you can, hold the position for a second, then slowly lower yourself back to the floor.

Gentle Crunches

If you can't manage either of the above stomach exercises, try this gentler alternative.

- Lie on the floor with your knees bent and your feet flat on the floor. Tilt your pelvis to protect your lower back from any strain.
- Tighten your stomach muscles, put your hands on your thighs and slowly lift your head up as high as you can to look at your knees, using your stomach muscles to lift you. Hold the position for a second, then lower yourself slowly back to the floor.

Pelvic Floor Exercises

If you're having a vaginal hysterectomy, get your pelvic floor muscles as fit as possible by doing pelvic floor exercises. You'll be advised to do them following the hysterectomy, but it's a good idea to start them before your operation, particularly if you are in line for vaginal repair (see page 19).

The pelvic floor muscles support the organs in your pelvic cavity. To find the right muscles, sit or lie comfortably with your knees slightly apart. Imagine you're trying to prevent a bowel movement; in order to do this, you must squeeze your muscles around your back passage.

Then imagine you're passing urine and want to stop the flow. To do this, you must also squeeze your muscles. You should be using the same group of muscles as before, but this exercise may seem harder. If you're unsure whether you're exercising the right muscles, slide a clean finger into your vagina and try the exercise. You should feel a gentle squeeze if you've got it right.

Next time you need to pass urine, try the exercise once its started to flow. Once you've stopped it, relax and empty your bladder. Don't hold your breath while you're doing it and don't worry if you can't stop it completely – your muscles will strengthen in time. Success won't happen overnight – it will take several weeks for muscles to become stronger and months before your muscles return to their former strength after the operation. Persevere – it will be worth it in the end.

- Slowly tighten and pull up the pelvic floor muscles as hard as you can and hold them tight for at least five seconds before relaxing.
- Pull up the muscles quickly and tightly, then relax immediately.
- Repeat both exercises at least five times.

As the muscles become stronger you'll be able to hold for longer than five seconds and do more repetitions. Then, do five fast and five slow exercises at least ten times a day.

The Power of Positive Thought

The majority of women I spoke to about their hysterectomy experiences had made an informed decision to have the operation, found out as much as they could beforehand and went into hospital with a positive attitude. It is surely no coincidence that most of them sailed through their operation and its aftermath with the minimum of complications. It could be argued that they were lucky, because there is no doubt that the attitude and the approach of the doctors and nurses treating you play an important part in determining whether or not your experience in hospital is positive or negative but how *you* approach the experience counts, too.

Joan recalls:

I'm a positive sort of person and I decided I was going to get through this with the minimum fuss and bother. Of course I was worried and nervous before I went in, because I'd been diagnosed as having micro-invasive cervical cancer, but I was determined not to let that get to me. I forced myself to get out of bed as quickly as I could and I discharged myself after three days, even though it had been an abdominal hysterectomy. Yet, I saw women on my ward who'd been in for a week and who didn't seem to be getting any better, and I suspect it was because they'd decided they were ill and were revelling in self-pity.

Relaxing Your Mind

Most of us are scared by the thought of operations and, in particular, anaesthesia. If you can learn a relaxation technique before you go into hospital, you'll be able to deal with the inevitable anxieties and stress more easily.

Hypnosis can be an effective form of relaxation if it's taught correctly. A hypnotic trance is an altered state of consciousness, a deep state of relaxation. Think about what it feels like when you're lying in bed half asleep and you want to go to the toilet, but you can't be bothered to get up because you don't want to upset that warm and wonderful feeling. That's pretty much what it feels like to be hypnotized.

Self-hypnosis is easily mastered, although it's best taught by a qualified hypnotherapist. It takes only a little daily practice to master the technique and, taught by a reputable hypnotherapist, it's completely safe. If you're in a light trance, you can come out of it any time you want.

A hypnotherapist may use a variety of techniques. You may be asked to concentrate on an image in your mind or to stare at a point on the ceiling until your eyes feel like closing. You might be asked to relax initially by clenching and unclenching various muscles until you can feel the tensions in your body disappear. Then you'll be talked down through the stages of hypnosis into a light trance.

Hypnotherapists often make tapes and these are useful while you're learning self-hypnosis. Played daily, you should get to the point when you relax when you hear the hypnotherapist's voice and then eventually you should find you don't need the tape at all.

If you can't get to a hypnotherapist, try this.

GETTING FIT FOR YOUR OPERATION

- Lie somewhere comfortable and shut your eyes, roll your eyeballs to the top of your head and then relax them.
- Slowly count from ten down to one, feeling tension disappearing from your body as you mentally count each number.
- When you get to one, imagine you're floating on a soft and fluffy cloud. Feel the cloud surrounding you with warmth and energy.
- Feel your body becoming lighter, warmer and more relaxed. You start to float upwards and you can feel yourself becoming weightless. You feel warm, relaxed, alert, healthy and calm. You feel great. Enjoy that feeling. Try to stay with it for as long as you can.
- When you want to come out of it, simply count up from one to ten, gradually becoming more alert with each number until you're wide awake by ten.

Another self-hypnosis technique is to lie in the 'corpse' position on the floor of a warm room.

- Lie on your back with your legs and arms slightly apart, palms facing upwards.
- Working from the feet upwards, tense and relax every part of your body in turn, finishing with your scalp and face.
- When you are deeply relaxed, start slowly breathing and counting rhythmically. Count from ten down to one. When you reach one, you should be in a light trance.
- Lie there for a few minutes, repeating to yourself, 'I am relaxed, I am happy, I am warm, I am safe, I am confident'. Feel the stress disappearing. Visualize yourself lying on a warm, golden, sandy beach with the waves lapping at your feet and the sun shining down on your body. Feel the warmth of the sun and lie there for as long as you want, letting these good and positive feelings wash over you. Visualize yourself not as a worried, anxious and stressed

person who is dreading going into hospital, but as a confident and relaxed individual who is looking forward to the hysterectomy, because afterwards you will feel a lot better. See yourself as that person, hold that image and feel good about it.
- When you count yourself out of your trance, say to yourself, 'When I have finished counting, I will be wide awake, full of life and happy and relaxed'.

If you spend half an hour a day practising self-hypnosis, you should become skilled enough to become very relaxed very quickly, whenever anxieties threaten to get the better of you.

Meditation

The main object of meditation is for you to learn to become master of your mind. If you suffer from stress and anxiety and cannot switch off, you have not achieved this – your mind has mastered you.

There are various forms of meditation, but they usually involve practising a series of techniques that calm your mind, change your awareness and bring your thoughts under control. Practising them regularly can bring significant health benefits. Clinical experiments have been performed on people who practise meditation, and they have been found to have a low pulse rate and oxygen consumption, less anxiety and increased concentration.

Meditation is simply learning the art of blocking out unpleasant and destructive thoughts and it takes many forms. Often the person is taught to focus on a word or mantra or an image, like a flickering candle. After a while, this leads the mind away from its normal thought processes and beyond.

To be able to meditate successfully, you need to practise daily for 10 to 15 minutes a time, each morning and night. Although it is best to learn from a teacher, there are some very good books that explain the techniques. However, you need to be highly motivated to teach yourself and it is probably easier to go to classes.

Try this.

- Sit in a chair or cross-legged on the floor, but don't lie down as you may fall asleep and it's essential you stay alert and wakeful.
- Ensure you won't be disturbed – take the phone off the hook.
- When you feel comfortable, close your eyes and take deep breaths. Feel your tensions slipping away. Focus your attention on a pleasant thought or the image of a flickering candle or a word or your breathing. Focusing your attention on something is a way of keeping out distractions.
- Start by focusing on the tip of your nose, then on the breath that is going into your nose and mouth, down your windpipe and into your lungs. Breathe slowly and deeply, and focus on your breathing for a while. Don't force it, let it happen.
- At first you'll find distractions keep flitting into your mind, trying to turn your attention away from the job in hand. Resist them and don't be dispirited if you can't concentrate. It takes a lot of practice before you can finally gain control of your mind.

Yoga

Yoga is an ancient system of spiritual development and at its highest level it is a form of meditation. However, it is also a very effective and enjoyable form of relaxation and exercise, and can help prevent illness and disease by keeping the body supple and maintaining bodily harmony.

Yoga concentrates on breathing, meditation and posture. A lot of attention is paid to breath control as practitioners of yoga believe that tension often results from incorrect, shallow breathing. Hatha yoga, the yoga most usually practised in the West, consists of a series of postures that you hold for as long as you feel comfortable.

The slow, controlled breathing yoga teaches, together with the postures, which keep the body flexible, tone up the internal organs, increase the circulation and have a calming effect on the body and mind. If you've never practised yoga before, it's best to go to a class to learn the basic postures, which can then be practised at home.

Find What's Best For You

While it's a good idea to learn some sort of relaxation technique, it's important that you find something you feel happy and comfortable with, rather than force yourself to do something you don't enjoy. But try to find some way of exercising your body and relaxing your mind that you do like before you have your hysterectomy as it should have a very beneficial effect on your physical and mental state and bolster your natural healing processes.

Chapter 6
IN HOSPITAL

Going into hospital for surgery can be a scary experience, especially if you've never been to hospital before. Huge, busy and with a characteristic smell that tends to linger, hospitals can seem strange and threatening places, and you're likely to feel even more anxious and apprehensive if you don't know what to expect. As you walk past wards and catch sight of patients who look very sick, you'll probably decide you'd rather be anywhere but there and have to summon up great reserves of courage to carry on. It helps, though, if you know exactly what's in store for you.

How the System Works

A consultant gynaecologist will probably have decided you needed a hysterectomy when you went for your appointment in outpatients. Unless your hysterectomy is for an urgent medical condition, such as invasive cancer – in which case you'll be admitted virtually immediately – you'll be put on a waiting list. You should receive a letter telling you your date of admission a few weeks in advance, although occasionally you might get a phone call from the hospital asking if you can come in at short notice because there has been a cancellation.

For those of us who have to organize jobs, children, pets and partners, this latter arrangement is not a practical proposition, but if you *can* manage to go in quickly, it has advantages in that it enables you to have your operation without a nail-biting, worrying wait.

If you tell your consultant you're willing to be a short-notice list patient, you'll virtually be on standby for the foreseeable future, and you're likely to get an early admission. You'll therefore need to have a bag permanently packed, leave a contact number where you can be reached any time and be ready to go as soon as you receive the call.

Sometimes your operation can be cancelled and your bed given to someone who has a more serious condition than yours if they're deemed to need immediate treatment. This is really bad luck and you have a right to know when you can get a new date.

Prior to your admission, the hospital should send you a letter with a list of things to take with you, such as:

- nightdresses
- dressing gown
- cardigan or bed jacket
- slippers
- toiletries
- towels
- hairbrush and comb
- pants
- sanitary pads (hospital ones are dire and there are never enough of them!).

Also take:

- coins for payphones
- writing paper, envelopes and stamps
- special treats, such as nice scent (a good morale booster)
- something to drink, such as fruit juice
- personal stereo
- some magazines.

Take cotton, rather than nylon nightdresses as hospitals are very hot places and if you wear nylon or most other man-made fibres, you'll quickly become uncomfortably sticky. There are no laundry facilities in hospitals, so if you haven't a partner or friend who can take your nightdresses away to wash, bring two or three.

Most hospitals have their own radios, but sometimes these have only a couple of channels and are not always reliable (the last time I was in hospital, the entire system had broken down), so take your own if you want to be on the safe side, as long as you've got an earpiece. If you're lucky enough to have a portable TV with an earpiece, take it – it'll save the inevitable arguments about which channels to watch in the hospital television room.

You'll need money for newspapers or anything else you might want to buy from the hospital shop. Don't take too much money or chequebooks or credit cards, because hospital lockers are not secure and even though most hospitals nowadays employ security staff, thefts do happen. Hand over any valuables to the nursing staff, who will put them in the hospital safe and give you a receipt. The same goes for jewellery: you may as well leave it at home as you won't be able to wear jewellery until after your operation, with the exception of your wedding ring, which a nurse will cover with tape.

I went into hospital with stacks of books on serious and heavy subjects, because I'd thought it would be an ideal opportunity to read all those books I'd always meant to. The books remained unopened and unread, because I found it so difficult to concentrate in hospital I could only cope with light reading. The sorts of books I usually buy at the airport to take on holiday were about all I could manage.

The nicest things I took with me were a single rose bud in a stem vase, which my husband had picked from the garden that morning, and a little bowl of pot pourri, the scent of which was a welcome relief from hospital smells. Touches of luxury such as expensive soap, fragrant body lotion or perfume make the experience a lot more bearable. A friend told me that the best investment she ever made was a crimson chiffon bed jacket to take into hospital, because she felt like a million dollars every time she put it on and was sure it hastened her recovery.

Each hospital's admissions procedure is different, but most will admit you the day before the operation as there are routine procedures and tests that need to be done beforehand.

Your first port of call will be the admissions desk, and it is here that you will go through the first of many wearisome routines – that of giving out your personal details. This is necessary because it is absolutely essential there is no confusion about your identity or your illness, so better to keep repeating yourself than end up having the wrong operation. Some hospitals now admit you on the ward itself to this end.

After you've been admitted, you may have to go to the pathology department to give a blood sample if you haven't already done so, in case you need a transfusion. Then you'll be shown to the bed you've been allocated on the ward.

Whether or not your stay in hospital is a good or a bad experience depends on the running of the hospital, your consultant, the nurses and the doctors. Being a patient in a hospital where the staff are prepared to be relaxed and accommodating about visiting times, and who are more concerned with your needs than sticking to hospital dogma, is a lot more pleasant than being in one that is run almost on army lines with no room to manoeuvre.

You're also going to sleep a lot easier if you've organized your domestic life before you're admitted, so you don't add to your anxieties by worrying about whether or not the dog's being taken for a walk every day or the kids will have someone to greet them when they get in from school. Some women spend the weeks before their admission stocking up the freezer with food for their husbands and children, which is a damning indictment on their husbands' ability to fend for themselves, but it does at least mean they can spend the duration of their stay in hospital secure in the knowledge that their families back home are getting fed.

The Nurses

Each ward is run by a sister (or charge nurse if he's a man) who is sometimes called a ward manager. Under her is a team of nurses, including usually a couple of staff nurses (RGN), who are fully qualified, and maybe some students, although most hospitals mainly train students in the classrooms nowadays. Healthcare assistants, or auxiliaries, have taken over a lot of the bedside nursing tasks the student nurses used to do.

A nurse will ask you to change into your night clothes, and you'll be given a plastic wrist bracelet on which is written your name, age, hospital number and the name of your surgeon. This cannot be removed without scissors, and it is essential that you do not try to remove it as this is the staff's confirmation that they've got the right person when you are unconscious. Without it, you may find yourself having your appendix, not your uterus taken out!

You should also be seen at some time by your own personal nurse – that is, a nurse who is responsible for looking after you during your stay. This is part of the Government's Patient's Charter, and is aimed at giving patients someone to whom they can personally relate during their time in hospital, rather than a succession of different faces. It's a great idea in theory, but, of course, nurses are not on duty 24 hours a day, so don't expect them to be on call whenever you want them. This nurse is responsible for your care plan, which you will be encouraged to be actively involved in.

A nurse will also come and take some personal details about you, including your religion, next of kin and any problems you might have regarding your home circumstances that might affect your stay. For example, if you are worrying because you've left an elderly relative at home, the hospital can arrange some sort of help for them with Social Services.

The nurse will ask you for a urine sample so that it can be tested to see if there is any infection, and also weigh you. This isn't so she can make you feel guilty about how overweight you are, it's so that the anaesthetist can work out how much anaesthetic you'll need. Your blood pressure and pulse will also be taken, and you may be given an ECG, if you are over 50 or there are doubts about your heart, or a chest X-ray.

The Doctors

The most junior doctor in 'the firm' under your consultant is called the house officer, and he or she will visit you and take a detailed medical history to determine your state of health. The house officer will want to know what medication, if any, you are taking, whether you have had any further symptoms since you were last seen by the consultant, if you have any known allergies and all about your past medical history and operations.

Some of the questions might not seem too relevant, but they all have a purpose. The object of them is to assess your current state of health and to discover whether or not there's anything the operating team needs to watch out for. You'll be asked to sign a consent form, and you should be quite clear about what you are consenting to.

Make sure you thoroughly discuss with your consultant exactly what sort of hysterectomy will be performed *before* you are admitted to hospital, be quite clear what will be removed and what will remain (see Chapter 4 for the terms used for the different types of hysterectomy) and make sure your wishes are included on the form. Some women have had oophorectomies (their ovaries removed) even though they did not consent to it, while others have had hysterectomies when they thought they were going in for a D & C. So, be absolutely sure that the operation stated on the consent form is the one you have made an informed decision to have. However, if a doctor thinks your life is in danger because of something they discover while you are in theatre, they can carry out virtually any surgical procedure on you while you are under anaesthetic. A surgeon can't wake you up if the operation isn't working and ask for your permission to try something else.

You should also be visited by the anaesthetist, who is responsible for keeping you alive during the operation. Most people's worries about operations centre on the anaesthetic. I know that whenever I have an anaesthetic there's the lurking thought in the back of my mind that I might not wake up, but, anaesthetics have never been safer and they have fewer side-effects than they used to. The risk of something going wrong is minimal.

The anaesthetist will want to know if you have any chest problems and you should say if you've ever suffered a bad reaction to anaesthesia before. Most people feel sick after an anaesthetic, and some are very sick indeed. Nowadays the anaesthetist can prescribe a drug that helps alleviate sickness or use a different sort of anaesthetic that has fewer side-effects if you're prone to sickness.

Some surgeons are starting to use spinal epidurals as well, so that the anaesthetic dose can be reduced and the after-effects lessened. A few women have had their entire hysterectomy performed while they were wide awake with only an epidural being administered and this may be an options if you can't tolerate anaesthesia for some reason.

Rachelle tells of her experience of this method:

A hysterectomy was suggested after I was diagnosed as having a very large fibroid which was causing me all manner of problems and it was too big to be removed any other way. But I've got a serious chest complaint which made a general anaesthetic risky, and so my surgeon said he'd do the operation with an epidural.

A green sheet was put up so I couldn't see what was going on. It took about half an hour and I couldn't feel a thing. They showed me the fibroid afterwards – it was enormous. I felt so well I was back at work as a hairdresser within three weeks.

The anaesthetist will talk to you about post-operative pain relief and ask you about dentures and crowns. Do remember to tell the anaesthetist about all your crowns, as you will have a tube inserted down your throat during your operation and care must be taken that any crowns are not dislodged.

A nurse will carry out pre-op procedures, such as shaving. Nowadays women are not shaved completely for an abdominal hysterectomy, just a strip at the top where the incision will be made. It needs to be done or it will get in the way as the incision is being stitched. Most hospitals let you do it rather than a nurse, but you may prefer to do it yourself in the comfort of your own bath the night before you're admitted.

You'll be asked to empty your bowels, and you may be given a suppository (a wax-like tube which is inserted into your rectum) or an enema. An enema is perfectly painless. A nurse inserts a syringe into your back passage and warm water is gently passed through. This ensures against accidents while you are on the operating table. You'll also be measured for special stockings which you must wear for a while after the operation, to help guard against blood clots and improve the circulation.

At midnight on the night before your operation, a sign will be hung above your bed saying 'Nil by mouth', and from then on you must have *nothing* to eat or drink – not even a sweet or a sip of water. If you feel desperately thirsty, you can rinse your mouth out with water, but otherwise nothing. If there is anything in your stomach during the operation, you may vomit while you're unconscious and choke.

On the Day

The morning of your operation, you are likely to feel frightened and nervous, especially if you have never had an operation before. You'll probably be visited by your consultant, or the senior registrar, for an encouraging last-minute chat. It can be reassuring to talk to other women on the ward who have had their hysterectomy, but sometimes it can make you feel worse! On any gynae ward, there's always one who can't wait to tell hair-raising tales about what could go wrong or to relate anecdotes about someone they know who's suffered every conceivable post-hysterectomy complication. When I was last in hospital, just before I went down to theatre, one of my fellow patients informed me that cockroaches had been found in the operating theatre the previous week, and I was only prevented from making a sharp exit by a nurse administering Valium. So the moral is, choose who you speak to with care!

You should remove all make-up, nail varnish and jewellery, and if you wear a wedding ring, it will be taped over. The nurse will tell you approximately what time your operation will be, and an hour or so before you're due to go down to theatre you'll be given a 'pre-med', which is usually a tranquillizer (often diazepam or temazepam) and it does make you feel a lot less tense – indeed, it can make you feel so happy you probably won't give two hoots about your impending op. It may even put you to sleep for a while. You'll also be given a drug that dries out the secretions in your nose and mouth.

You'll be given a theatre gown and hat to wear, and when the time comes for you to be taken to the theatre, two porters will arrive, transfer you on to a trolley and wheel you down to the theatre with a nurse. As you leave the ward, your identity and what operation you'll be having will be checked and it will be checked again when you reach the anaesthetics room.

At this point, your nurse will hand you over to the theatre nurse, who is usually a kindly and reassuring soul, as this is an anxious time for most patients. ECG pads will probably be attached to your chest so your heart can be monitored and the anaesthetist will then insert a needle into a vein in your hand and ask you to count to ten while the anaesthetic is being administered. This is the time I want to make my excuses and leave, but in the space of five to eight seconds you'll be unconscious and know no more. A tip: if the anaesthetic is passed too quickly into your vein, unconsciousness is terrifyingly fast. If you, like me, prefer it to be a little more gentle, ask the anaesthetist to administer it more slowly.

Once you're unconscious, you'll be put on a variety of machines that make up your life support system during the operation. Your heart, blood pressure and pulse will be monitored constantly, your breathing will be done for you by a ventilator, and a cuff on the tube inserted down your throat is inflated at the bottom of your windpipe to ensure that no secretions get into your lungs.

When You Wake Up

How long the operation takes depends on what sort of hysterectomy you are having. A traditional abdominal hysterectomy can take as little as 30 minutes, whereas a laparoscopic hysterectomy can take a couple of hours or more. Once the operation is completed, you'll be taken to the recovery room, where the tube in your throat will be removed and you'll start to breathe normally.

You'll be given some sort of analgesia to relieve the pain, and a nurse will stay with you until you have recovered sufficiently to be taken back to the ward. You'll probably wake to the nurse calling your name, and there may be an oxygen mask over your face. Regular blood pressure and pulse checks will be made until you wake up. Some people don't remember this time and don't really wake up until they are back on the ward.

Fear of the unknown means you spend a lot of time worrying needlessly, so it helps if you know what might be in store for you when you do come round. If you've had an abdominal hysterectomy, you're likely to spend much of the 18 hours after your operation drifting in and out of sleep, and you probably won't come to properly until the following day. Your throat may well feel sore where the tube has been and, although your wound may feel tender, you shouldn't be in pain because you'll have been given painkillers. You might feel a tightness in your chest and want to cough, and if you can, do so – it'll help prevent the possibility of a chest infection.

You might wake up from your operation with a drain, drip or catheter attached (or even all three). If this happens to you, don't be alarmed – they look far worse than they are. Not everyone will have one or all of them, but knowing that you might means it's less of a shock if you do.

A Drip

A drip is a salt and sugar solution in a clear bag that is hung up on a stand. The solution is dripped into you through a tube taped to the back of your hand via a needle passed into a vein. After an operation, you are likely to be very dehydrated, and you'll be unable to eat for a while. The anaesthetic may well make you feel sick. Eventually you'll be allowed sips of water, but you probably won't be allowed anything more than a cup of tea until the following day – if that. A drip ensures you don't dehydrate.

A Catheter

A catheter is a thin tube that is inserted into the urethra (the tube that carries the urine out of the body) to draw the urine from the bladder into a bag. It's inserted during the operation and sometimes it's left in place for a while afterwards, because the bladder can take a bit of time to function on its own. It's usually removed within 24 hours after an abdominal hysterectomy if all is well, but after a vaginal hysterectomy it may be left there for a while longer. If you haven't had a catheter and you can't pass water by the following morning, one may well be put in. It does feel as if you're passing water the whole time, but, although it can be a bit uncomfortable, it shouldn't be painful.

A Drain

A drain is a tube that leads from the wound to a little bottle at the other end and it allows any blood or tissue fragments that might have been left behind to drain out of the wound. As soon as the wound starts to heal, it stops oozing and the drain is removed (usually three or four days later). Drains look pretty horrible, but they're painless.

Discharge

You'll have a brownish vaginal discharge after the operation, but the nurses will have put a pad in place while you were unconscious. It might be streaked with blue, but don't worry – this is an antiseptic dye that's been used to sterilize your vagina. The time to start worrying is:

- if the discharge becomes bright red, heavy or contains clots as this may be an indication of internal bleeding (secondary haemorrhage)
- if it becomes offensive or smelly, as this could denote an infection.

If either of these things happen, tell the nurse, *at once*.

Other Things to Know About

A physiotherapist may visit you the morning after your operation and encourage you to cough gently, but you'll probably feel the need to do so anyway. The most comfortable way of coughing is to sit up in bed, bend your knees and either put your arms or a pillow over the wound before you cough. If you've had a vaginal hysterectomy, put your hand over your pad and then cough. The physiotherapist will also show you some simple exercises to do, which will start your stomach muscles working again.

As soon as you open your eyes, concentrate on keeping your legs moving. Start by wriggling your toes up and down and then clench and unclench your calf muscles, but don't cross your legs. Flex your feet up and down at the ankle. Taking three or four deep breaths regularly helps expel any remaining anaesthetic from your system. Do this as soon as you wake up, and carry on doing it even when you're up and about.

Keeping your legs moving until you can get out of bed is essential to help reduce the risk of chest infections or, more seriously, deep-vein thrombosis (DVT). A DVT is when a blood clot forms in the veins of the legs, which can occasionally happen if you're in bed for any length of time as the blood flow in the legs slows. This can be life-threatening. If the clot breaks off, it is carried along in the general blood circulation and the danger then is that it might not be able to pass through the arteries. When a broken-off piece of clot blocks the pulmonary artery that leads to the lungs, it's known as a pulmonary embolism. This is a not uncommon post-operative complication and can be fatal. Surgery and anaesthetics increase the risk, which is why the nursing staff are anxious to get you up and out of bed as quickly as possible and may give you DVT stockings to wear.

If a thrombosis occurs in the deep veins of the leg, it becomes painful and swollen as fluid builds up at the site of the blockage. A pulmonary embolism can cause chest pain and breathlessness. If you have any pain in your leg or chest or any shortness of breath, *tell the nurse immediately*. Anticlotting drugs can quickly dissolve the blockage as soon as it's diagnosed, but it's vital it's caught in time.

Getting your blood circulating normally is the main reason the nursing staff want you out of bed and walking the day after your operation, and they generally combine this with another necessity – getting you to go to the lavatory. Walking to the lavatory may seem an impossible task, but, with the support of a nurse, you should be able to do it. An incentive is that most people find it absolutely impossible to wee into a bedpan! Once you get yourself moving, you should find yourself becoming mobile again quicker than you'd imagined, but don't overdo it – rest is also part of the healing process. You'll feel very tired, so listen to your body. If you've had a vaginal or laparoscopic hysterectomy, you'll undoubtedly recover a lot more quickly and have fewer after-effects than if you've had an abdominal hysterectomy.

For a week or so after the operation, you'll probably worry like mad about your stitches bursting, especially if you cough or laugh, but they won't. You'll probably get used to moving around with one hand supporting the wound. It gives you security and makes you feel more comfortable, but there's no need to worry about the wound coming adrift even if you vomit, which puts a lot of strain on the stomach muscles.

Most of us want to rocket around as though nothing had happened, but it doesn't take long to realize that moving about requires some skill and technique because you're likely to be stiff and sore. Getting out of bed is the first challenge. Bend your knees upwards and roll sideways towards the edge of the bed, keeping your legs bent together. Let your legs swing to the floor as you sit up, supporting yourself with an elbow and a hand. Reverse this process when you want to get back into bed.

If you are attached to a drip or drain, which makes moving about difficult (try washing your hair with a drip in!), you'll find you manage to adapt. Most hospitals serve meals at a communal table for everyone who isn't confined to bed, and it'll make you feel a lot better if you can get up and talk to people.

It can be hard to eat for as long as three days afterwards. Janet found this:

Every time I smelled food I felt ill. Three days later, when I did start fancying food again, I took one look at what they served up and thought, forget it! I asked my husband to bring in things I really fancied and that were good for me, like fresh fruit and nice cheeses, and that was how I managed to start eating.

When you have abdominal surgery, your intestines are handled and this can affect the bowels, particularly as you haven't eaten for a couple of days. The problem can be worsened if you had adhesions or old scar tissue that caused your pelvic organs to stick to your intestines so that they needed to be carefully separated during the operation.

Normally, waste products are pushed along the intestines and out of the body by a constant series of spasm-like movements called peristalsis. Abdominal surgery can stop this working normally, causing gases to build up because they cannot escape until the bowel is working properly again – which often doesn't happen until the third or fourth day after the operation.

Wind is normally regarded as a bit of a joke, but it's anything but amusing and can be very painful, particularly if you get 'referred' pain under the shoulders caused by the accumulation of wind in the abdomen. The nurses can give you a peppermint remedy to relieve it, and Lucozade and soda works well. All this means, of course, that when your system *does* start working normally, you can get some highly embarrassing moments if you pass wind inadvertently. The embarrassment tends to pass quickly as the other patients on the ward are in the same situation as you, and you soon learn to see the funny side of it.

The nursing staff will be monitoring you to see whether or not you have emptied your bowels. The more you move about, the quicker things will start working again, but some people need a laxative to set things moving.

Occasionally, if there has been extensive handling of the intestines, they can go into spasm afterwards and cause an obstruction in the bowel. This means you will not be able to rid your body of its waste and soon you'll start to feel very ill indeed. The first signs are loss of appetite, colicky pains that get worse and worse, then you'll probably start vomiting. You may well have been discharged by the time this happens as often the symptoms don't appear for a week after the operation. If this is the case, contact your GP immediately.

You'll probably be sent back to hospital for an X-ray to confirm that there is an obstruction. If that's the problem, a tube will probably be inserted through your nose and down into your stomach to drain it of its contents, and a drip will be put into your hand to ensure you do not get dehydrated. Giving the intestines a chance to rest usually gets them working again. You'll know when things are getting back to normal when you can pass wind, but, very occasionally, surgery might be needed.

If you've had an abdominal hysterectomy, the dressing is usually removed from the wound on about the third day. The incision will be held together with stitches or clips, and these will usually be removed by a nurse about five days after the operation or whenever the wound has healed. Clips sometimes hurt a little when they are removed, especially if they are deeply embedded, and even stitches can hurt if the skin has grown over them. If you have had a vaginal hysterectomy, you will have no external stitches.

Exercises to do After Your Operation

Pelvic Floor Exercises

As we saw earlier, the pelvic floor muscles are like a sort of sling that supports the organs in your pelvic cavity. Ideally, they should be taut. When your uterus has been removed, the surgery may affect these muscles, which still have to support the vagina, anus and urethra. If they are weak, it can lead to incontinence and even prolapse – even if you've had a hysterectomy. Pelvic floor exercises can tone up your muscles and make them strong enough to support your abdominal organs efficiently. Check with your doctor how soon after your operation you can practise pelvic floor exercises.

Hopefully you will have been doing these exercises before your operation, particularly if you have had a prolapse (see pages 18–19), but, if not, see pages 62–63 to find the right muscles as it's important to work these specific muscles for the exercises to have the desired effect.

- Draw up and squeeze all the pelvic floor muscles.
- Hold that squeeze for five seconds, then slowly let go. Don't hold your breath as you do this.
- Repeat four times an hour or as often as you can.

If you get into the habit of practising pelvic floor exercises as part of your daily routine, it will help you guard against incontinence.

Stomach Muscle Exercises

You'll probably feel as though your stomach muscles have vanished if you've had an abdominal hysterectomy, but if you worked hard on building up your stomach muscles before you went into hospital (see pages 60–1), it shouldn't take long to get them back into shape again. You won't be up to much at first, but some gentle abdominal exercises will help strengthen them. The hospital physiotherapist will probably give you some exercises to do, which are variations on the following.

Pelvic Tilts
- Lie on your back with a pillow under your head and your knees bent up and together, your feet on the mattress.
- Pull your stomach muscles in and slightly tilt your bottom upwards, tilting your pelvis in towards your navel and stretching your lower back.
- Then, press your lower back down into the mattress, without holding your breath.
- Hold the position for five seconds, then relax.
- Repeat six times, three times a day.

Knee Rolls
- Lie flat on your back with knees bent up and together.
- Pull your stomach muscles in and let your knees gently drop to the left as far as you can (which probably won't be very far at first, but you should be able to go further and further each day), then raise them and lower them to the right.
- Don't hold your breath as you do this.
- Repeat six times, three times a day.

Tummy Tightener

- Lie on your back, pull in your stomach muscles as much as you can and hold them tight for a count of four. Don't hold your breath.
- Repeat six times, three times a day. Don't worry if you can't do it at first – you should see a marked improvement every day.

Head Lifts

- Lie on your back with your head on a pillow, your knees bent up and your feet flat on the mattress.
- Tuck your chin in to your chest, put your hands on your thighs, tighten your stomach muscles, then slowly raise your head towards your knees.
- Hold the position, without holding your breath, while you slowly count to five, then relax.
- Repeat six times, three times a day.

A variation on this is to lift your head, tuck your chin in and, with your right arm straight, reach over to touch your left thigh or knee. Relax, and repeat on the opposite side three times each side, six times a day.

The Blues

It's common to feel weepy, depressed, emotional and very vulnerable after any operation, but these feelings can be more acute after a hysterectomy because many women suffer a profound feeling of loss. More about this in Chapter 9, but just to say here that it's absolutely normal to feel like this. Before the operation, you will probably have been very anxious and worried, and maybe started to be aware of your own mortality. The relief that it's over, delayed shock, the fact that your hormones may be all over the place, plus your being vulnerable and absolutely dependent on others all contribute to post-operative depression. It *is* depressing and frustrating to feel physically weak and feeble, especially if you're normally a fit and active person.

As you start to feel better, you'll be left on your own more and more, and you won't receive so much obvious care from the nurses. The realization that you've got to stand on your own feet and take charge of your own recovery, even though you still feel weak and vulnerable, can make you feel depressed. Sometimes there's no obvious reason for your feeling the way you do, it just happens. Talking helps, either to your fellow patients or to your nurse.

Janet remembers:

There were a lot of mixed emotions when I had my hysterectomy. Nobody talked to me about it – my doctor just fobbed me off with hormones and I realize now that a lot of the depression I suffered afterwards, which I'd put down to a surgical menopause, was all to do with the sadness I felt about losing my womb. It was a weird feeling. Part of you is gone and you don't know why – it's like having a baby, part of you's sad and weepy but the other part is happy. The difference is, you don't have that happy part. I cried ever such a lot. I'd always imagined myself with a large family, and there I was in my early thirties with no possibility of having any more babies. I always say think hard before having a hysterectomy, it does change you. If you can live with what's wrong with you, do so.

Visitors

In theory, having visitors is wonderful. Before you go into hospital, you'll probably ask all and sundry to drop in, and plan the duration of your stay like a social occasion. The reality is, if you've had an abdominal hysterectomy, for the first two days at least after the operation, you probably won't feel like seeing anyone other than your partner, because you won't have the energy or the inclination to make conversation. Most hospitals have long and flexible visiting hours and it can be tiring if you have loads of visitors, particularly if they include children. Nurses are watchful on such occasions and if you look particularly tired they often tactfully suggest to your visitors that you need a rest. Keep your visitors to a minimum. You'll be glad you did.

Complications

Most people come through their operations without having any problems, but occasionally there can be complications afterwards such as:

- a urinary infection, which manifests itself as a burning pain when you pass water
- a haematoma – a blood clot that can form in the wound if blood leaks into the tissues and looks like a bruise under the skin (if it's large, it will need to be drained)
- constipation, which can be eased by laxatives
- infection of the wound – if the wound turns an angry red colour and pus appears, this suggests that there is an infection, which can be serious if it's ignored
- wound abscess, which can develop if bacteria gets into the wound
- vaginal bleeding (see pages 97–8).

Chapter 7
GOING HOME

Most people leave hospital with mixed feelings. On the one hand it's wonderful to be going home, with the anxieties that built up as you waited to go into hospital behind you. On the other hand, you're likely to feel insecure and vulnerable. While you've been in hospital, your every need has been met and you've been protected, cared for and fussed over. You've had no responsibilities, you haven't had to think for yourself and you've felt utterly safe. Now you've got to manage alone, and even for those with a supportive partner or family or friends, the prospect can be daunting. Without some sort of support, it's a nightmare. If you've had an abdominal hysterectomy, there's no way you'll be able to look after yourself alone for a week or so afterwards.

When you leave depends on how quickly you heal, what sort of operation you've had, the skill of your surgeon, your state of mind and what sort of back-up arrangements you have at home. Most patients leave hospital five to seven days after an abdominal hysterectomy, and three to four days after a vaginal or laparoscopic hysterectomy. But when you leave also depends on *you* and what you feel like. Don't be pushed out if you don't feel up to it. If you feel shaky or unwell or you're not sure you're going to be able to manage, say so. They're not going to throw you out on to the streets if you feel you can't cope.

When you're discharged, you should be told when to return for a check-up in the out-patients clinic, and the kindly nurses will give you reassuring information about how you're likely to feel over the next few days and what to expect. You may be given some notes about exercises and dos and don'ts – things you should and shouldn't do. You'll also be given a letter for your GP and any medication you may need, and you should take your discharge letter to your GP as soon as possible. If you've had problems with your wound healing and are being discharged with a dressing, you may need referring to a district nurse to have the dressing changed.

Joan remembers how she felt when she came to leave hospital:

After I had a run in with the sister, who insisted on treating me like a six-year-old, I thought, I've got to get out of this place. So, I called my friend I was due to go and stay with when I left hospital and she collected me, four days after my operation for cervical cancer. I felt marvellous physically but mentally very weepy – I missed my dad, who's been dead some years, and I missed having a mother. Not my mother, because she and I never got on, just a mother figure to care for me because I felt very vulnerable. You're not in control and I felt very nervous about trusting others to care for me, and, as well as that, I had lingering worries that the cancer might return. I felt a little unloved and really felt the absence of a regular partner.

Leaving hospital can be a bewildering experience. After a week of being cocooned from the rough and tumble of everyday living, you're likely to emerge blinking and disorientated into the outside world. Walking down the ward might have been a breeze, but walking through the hospital to your waiting car or taxi outside may well seem like a marathon. Much has to do with the anaesthetic, the effects of which will stay with you for a few weeks, depending on what sort of operation you have had.

The after-effects of a vaginal or laparoscopic hysterectomy are far less than those of an abdominal hysterectomy, which tends to leave you feeling extremely tired and leaden-legged – something you don't notice while you're in hospital. Let's assume you've had an abdominal hysterectomy.

The First Fortnight

You should do absolutely nothing for the first five days, and rest each day for at least an hour. In practice, you'll probably find you spend most of the day reading or watching TV and drifting in and out of sleep as a result. It's important you have some sort of support, from a partner, friends or neighbours, for a couple of weeks after the operation – ideally people who are sensitive enough to realize that you need time alone while you convalesce and that too much talking is very tiring indeed.

Some hospitals can arrange for you to spend this fortnight in a convalescence home, especially if you have no support system at home, although cutbacks have made this a rare luxury nowadays. Those of us with families at home would probably rather stay at home with them than be cared for by strangers in a convalescence home, although such a break can ensure that when you do return to your home routine, you're fit enough to cope. In practice, most local authorities' budgets do not stretch to being able to send even very needy patients to convalescence homes, but if you can afford it, it can be worthwhile.

The advantage of going to a convalescence home is that you can get through the two weeks following your operation under the watchful eye of experienced staff without having to cope with the demands and stresses of everyday life. Those two weeks are usually the worst because you're likely to feel very tired, confused and disorientated, and quite unable to cope with minor domestic crises.

Sarah tells of her experience:

Two weeks after my op, I was at home alone when someone left the gate open and the dog went charging off down the road barking at someone. My automatic reflex was to run after him and of course I couldn't. So, I propped myself up at the kitchen door and tried shouting and nothing happened. My voice came out in a croaky whisper and it seemed weeks before I could start bellowing at the kids and the dog again. It was my stomach muscles, they were shot to pieces. You don't realize until such occasions what a wide variety of tasks your stomach muscles perform. I've no stomach muscles now, just a wedge of flab, and nothing I can do will shift it.

This is a very frustrating time because you're desperate to be better and you actually *feel* better until you try to do something and you find you're not. This can make you feel rather crotchety. You'll be able to walk up and down stairs, but you'll probably need a rail to hang on to for a while, and you won't be able to spend long on your feet for that first couple of weeks. You may well need to support yourself when you stand up as well. Don't be surprised if you keep dropping off to sleep at odd hours of the day either, especially if you've overexerted yourself.

Joan remembers:

I got so fed up during those weeks afterwards I'd cry with frustration. It was bad enough that I felt so weak – and before then I'd been going to a gym three times a week and I was really fit – but my mind seemed to have gone as well. I'm a journalist and I thought I'd be able to work at home, but I couldn't think straight, couldn't read a book of any seriousness, couldn't even read a newspaper other than a tabloid. I seemed to stay brain-dead for about a month afterwards. There were times when I thought I'd never get better.

There are no hard and fast rules about how quickly you should convalesce and you should take it gently, one step at a time, paying special attention to what your body is telling you. Much depends on how young and fit you were before you went in, and how much anaesthetic you've had. Janet worked as a cleaner and it was six months before she felt fit enough to work again, but Joan felt well enough to return to her job as a journalist after two months.

One Step at a Time

You may feel like having a slow walk on the sixth or seventh day, and if that feels comfortable, gradually increase the distance you walk on subsequent days and rest if you feel tired. You won't be able to lift a kettle of water until at least the third week, and only do so then if you can do it comfortably and without pain. After a month, you might feel well enough do light housework, such as washing-up, dusting or light shopping, but don't attempt hoovering until the fifth or sixth week.

Be careful about driving a car. The after-effects of anaesthetics can linger, so, if you've had an abdominal hysterectomy, don't attempt to drive until at least a month afterwards, and then only do so if you feel absolutely happy and confident. Just to be on the safe side, take another driver with you the first couple of times. Most women are not as fortunate as Mr Cheng Lee's patient, who, you will recall, felt she could have driven herself home from hospital 24 hours after her hysterectomy (see page 52).

Joan remembers the first time she drove after her operation:

Four weeks after my hysterectomy, the friend I was staying with became ill and I had no option but to drive into town to pick up her prescription for her. Driving was just about all right as I took it carefully, but, then, would you believe it, I hadn't gone far, when I

> *got a puncture. Normally I can change a wheel, but there was absolutely no way I could even contemplate doing it. I had to flag down a man and ask him to do it, which I hated doing, but, fortunately, he was very nice and understanding about it.*

Try not to bend or lift anything for at least a month after the operation or, if you need to bend, bend at the knees, keeping your back straight. You shouldn't attempt to lift anything heavy or move furniture around until at least 12 weeks after your hysterectomy, because internal stitches need a chance to heal. Take care if you've got small children – picking them up is usually a reflex action, but, if you do, you could end up doing yourself great damage. You should be able to go swimming after four to six weeks.

When you go to see your gynaecologist for your six-week check-up, you should be feeling almost back to normal, although maybe still tired. It can be frustrating to realize you're still not 100 per cent fit by then because most people believe they will be after this time, but, alas, it's sometimes not the case after an abdominal hysterectomy. It can be very depressing as week after week goes by and you still don't feel right, particularly if you've always been a very active person, but take heart. The day will come when you get out of bed and suddenly realize you feel great. It'll probably happen like a bolt from the blue, but, when it does, that realization acts like a tonic, lifting your spirits more than any stimulant can.

Hygiene

After a hysterectomy – or indeed any surgical procedure involving the genital area – it's important to be scrupulously clean to minimize the risk of infection. Have a bath each day and pay special attention to cleaning your genital area, but don't use a douche.

Vitamin Supplements

You can hasten your recovery by eating a well-balanced, nutritious diet, one that is high in fibre and includes plenty of fresh fruit and vegetables (see Chapter 5). Your immune system has got its work cut out during this post-operative healing period, and this is the one time most doctors agree that taking vitamin supplements is a good idea.

Vitamin and mineral supplements are no substitutes for a nutritious diet, however, so if you eat junk food but think you can make up for it by taking supplements, you'll be disappointed. Normally you shouldn't need supplements at all if you are eating well and exercising, but after surgery, your body's defences will need a bit of a boost to get you healthy again and help fight off infection.

A lot of research has been done the results of which suggest that taking supplements of the antioxidant nutrients, as well as eating a nutritious diet, can boost the immune system and help protect us against various diseases. A high intake of vitamin E has been found to increase the body's immune response, vitamin C and selenium enhance the immune system, and vitamin A stimulates the immune response and controls the growth of body tissues. Vitamin E is found in green leafy vegetables, nut oils and cereals, and vitamin C is found in rosehips, blackcurrants and citrus fruits but you'd need to eat huge amounts of all these in order to raise your vitamin intake appreciably.

So, taking vitamin supplements after surgery can promote faster healing, but beware. Indiscriminate taking of vitamins can lead to an imbalance (some vitamins only work in conjunction with others, for example) and some (notably vitamin A) can actually be toxic if taken in excessive quantities. A good multivitamin and mineral supplement is the safest to take unsupervised.

Evening Primrose Oil

Evening primrose oil belongs to a group of vitamin-like substances known as essential fatty acids (EFAs). EFAs cannot be made by the body – they must be provided by the diet. They form part of every single cell membrane and are involved in almost every biological function. Without the support, strength and flexibility they give to cell membranes, skin would sag and age, nails flake and break and hair would become dull and dry. But, to be of any value, EFAs have to be converted into *other* fatty acids, such as gammalinolenic acid (GLA) – a powerful, active ingredient that is found in evening primrose oil – and, finally, into prostaglandins, which are active fighters in the immune system's operation.

Scientists are still trying to understand the precise role EFAs play in the functioning of the immune system, but what they have discovered is that when there is a deficiency, the production of T cells is impaired, making us more susceptible to infection.

What is starting to become accepted is that evening primrose oil can play an important part in treating a number of disorders, especially menstrual problems. There is also a school of thought that believes the GLA found in evening primrose oil may be able to protect us from infection. EFAs in sufficient quantities can fight viruses, so it seems as though evening primrose oil can play an important part in enhancing immune function. Taking 1000 mg a day will help your natural healing processes.

Bleeding

Vaginal bleeding or a discharge can be very scary in the weeks following a hysterectomy. It's easy to think something's wrong, but it's usually only internal dissolving stitches and the body's way of cleaning out the system after the disruption of the operation.

The discharge may be brownish, yellowy or slightly blood-stained, but it should stop after two or three weeks. Wear a pad rather than a tampon, because of the risk of infection if you use a tampon, and change pads regularly. If the discharge is foul-smelling, it may mean there's some sort of infection, and if you start to bleed heavily and the blood is bright red, see your GP *at once*. You should also see your GP if your discharge or bleeding goes on longer than three weeks, as it could be a sign that something's wrong.

Putting on Weight

A hysterectomy, in itself, should not cause you to put on weight, particularly if you try to eat healthily and take gentle exercise in ever-increasing amounts. The only reason you may start piling on the pounds is if you're at all predisposed to do so, because you're going to be inactive for a while and not sticking to any sort of routine, and when that happens it's easy to get into a snacking habit. You put on weight, after all, when your calorie intake is more than the calories you use up, and if you're sitting about for most of the time you're not using up many calories.

Thinking about controlling your calorie intake is the last thing you'll want to do after a major operation when you're probably feeling a bit sorry for yourself or you're bored out of your mind. You're more like to want to comfort eat as a result. A friend of mine found herself uncontrollably cramming after dinner mints into her mouth every time she sat down.

Resist the lure of food, though. If you must comfort eat, keep a fridge full of celery and carrot sticks to eat with a fromage frais dip. It'll give you something to stick in your mouth, fill you up, and prevent you from putting on weight. If you do put on a lot of weight following your op, you'll find it difficult to get your stomach muscles working again.

Self-help Groups

It can be very useful to be in touch with a hysterectomy support group. It's reassuring and supportive to be in touch with people who have had direct experience of the sorts of problems you may be experiencing, and it can make you feel a lot less isolated. Even better, get in touch with a support group *before* you go into hospital. There'll be a lot of fears you'll want allayed and questions you'll want answered.

You may also feel like talking to a counsellor who is experienced in dealing with hysterectomy patients before and after your operation. Hysterectomy counselling is not usually offered by hospitals, although some have set up pre-operative support groups where women due to have an operation are invited to meet gynae nurses or nurse/counsellors who can answer their questions and quell any anxieties they might have.

The more information you have, the less nervous you'll be when you have your operation.

You'll find the address of the Hysterectomy Support Network in the Useful Addresses section, and this organization has a wide-ranging list of contacts, but there are other local groups as well. Your GP or ward sister should also be able to help.

Back to Work

When you go back to work depends entirely on how you feel – there's no set time. Many firms expect to see you back within six to eight weeks, but it's important that you go back when you feel 100 per cent fit, which you may not be after this time. Go back before you feel ready, and you're likely to have a set-back. The best option of all is if you can go back to work part time, so you can slowly acclimatize yourself to the unfamiliar (and very tiring) routine of working again.

If you've had a laparoscopic hysterectomy, you may feel fit enough to go back to work within a month. If you've had an abdominal hysterectomy, you may not feel up to working for three months. Much depends, too, on what sort of job you do. Janet had worked cleaning newly built houses before her operation, a job that involved a lot of lifting, stretching and hard physical labour, and she wasn't able to work again for six months, although the consultant had told her she'd be ready to go back to work after *three* months. If your job involves you sitting at a desk all day, you'll probably go back to work sooner than if you spend most of your working day standing on your feet. Listen to your body, too, whatever work you do, and return to work when it tells you to.

Chapter 8
HYSTERECTOMY, HORMONES AND HRT

Surgeons often think that once a woman is past the menopause and therefore doesn't 'need' her ovaries any longer, they might as well remove them to guard against the fairly small possibility of her developing ovarian cancer in the future. This is a very debatable decision and one that should not be taken without a thorough discussion with the woman concerned (see Chapter 4). Although the effects of removing the ovaries on a post-menopausal woman are nothing like as drastic as they are if the woman is pre-menopausal, nevertheless, there will be a difference. The ovaries are responsible for a number of important hormones, some of which go on being produced even after the menopause.

Natural and Surgical Menopause

Hormones are the body's chemical messengers. They're produced by different glands in the body and are circulated round the body in the bloodstream. Their output is controlled by a part of the brain called the hypothalamus and they play an important part in the mental and physical workings of our bodies, and also our sexuality.

During the menstrual cycle, our ovaries produce the hormones oestrogen and progesterone in amounts that vary according to which phase of the cycle we are in. As well as large amounts of these female hormones, the ovaries also produce small amounts of testosterone and other male hormones. These hormones do not work in isolation: testosterone, for example, works with oestrogen to give us our sex drive.

A natural menopause takes place over a number of years. As the reproductive system gradually winds down, the ovaries shrivel and generate less and less oestrogen, although they still carry on producing *small* quantities of oestrogen and male hormones for some years after the menopause. If you've had your uterus removed but not your ovaries, you'll have a natural menopause. If you've had your uterus *and* your ovaries removed, though, you'll have a surgical menopause because this hormone supply is withdrawn immediately, and the body has no time to adjust to the loss. If HRT isn't given, the effects can be severe, as Janet found:

> *I couldn't think straight, couldn't do anything. Three months after my hysterectomy, I thought I was having a nervous breakdown, so I went to see my GP, who discovered I hadn't been given HRT implants as is normal for someone of my age – 33 – and I was in a sudden menopause. My GP put me on Premarin 625, which made me feel a bit better, but I still didn't feel right, so he upped the dose and I lost all sexual feelings, I was permanently tired, I had hot flushes, depression and felt so miserable. My head felt as though it was somewhere else.*

Other side-effects that can follow a surgical menopause are vaginal dryness, weight gain, headaches, backache and a very real loss of sex drive. This is why surgeons recommend HRT for women who experience a surgical menopause after their hysterectomy, or to treat natural menopausal symptoms.

HRT is merely the replacement of the oestrogen that's been lost. Contrary to what the tabloid press would sometimes have us believe, it is not a cure-all, nor a rejuvenator, although it can improve the texture and bloom of the skin and it does seem to alleviate psychological symptoms and go hand in hand with increased energy. What it *does* definitely do is reverse the effects of the menopause, but its greatest advantage is that it also helps protect against osteoporosis, heart disease and stroke.

Hot Flushes and Night Sweats

These are the commonest symptoms of a surgical (and natural) menopause and doctors don't really know why they happen, other than that the abrupt withdrawal of oestrogen can affect the body's temperature control mechanism.

Hot flushes can occur dozens of times a day and, although they don't usually last long, they can be uncomfortable and embarrassing. Most women experience little more than a 30-second warm blush that spreads from the neck upwards, but for some the flushes last for 2 or 3 minutes and are accompanied by drenching perspiration and palpitations.

Night sweats are ghastly. Most women who've experienced them speak of waking up in the night with their nightdresses and sheets literally soaked.

Vaginal Dryness

Oestrogen is responsible for the lubrication secreted by the vaginal walls when you are sexually aroused. Without it your vagina can become uncomfortably dry, the lining thinner and the glands producing fewer secretions, resulting in pain and soreness when you make love. The vagina is also more prone to infections if it is dry, itchy or irritated, as it can tear easily.

HRT stimulates the production of vaginal secretions, but there is a natural and much more enjoyable way to increase your vaginal secretions – make love more frequently. This stimulates the glands to produce more lubricating secretions.

Incontinence

Incontinence can often follow the menopause as the bladder muscles can become slack due to lack of oestrogen, but it can also result from having had a difficult labour. Even mild incontinence can mean you leak urine when coughing, sneezing or exercising.

Practising pelvic floor exercises should ensure you keep your muscles toned, and HRT should help if symptoms are severe.

Psychological Symptoms

These are often the worst to deal with and include depression, forgetfulness, confusion, feelings of unreality rather like a panic attack, poor memory, inability to concentrate, general feeling of unwellness, tiredness and lack of energy.

HRT really can make a difference to these sorts of symptoms and abolish them almost at a stroke.

Who's at Risk?

Research has shown that those most likely to suffer menopausal problems acutely are:

- women who have had an early menopause, particularly a surgical one
- smokers and excessive drinkers, because this can affect the ovaries' oestrogen output
- women who have suffered from PMS may experience worse

psychological symptoms
- thin women, who have fewer reserves of oestrogen (the fatter you are, the more oestrogen you have naturally in your body).

Osteoporosis

Osteoporosis is a chronic, degenerative disease that has become so common it is reaching epidemic proportions among older people, mostly women. Although it doesn't kill directly, it can lead to such a physical deterioration that death can occur from related conditions, and it's associated with oestrogen and calcium deficiency.

Osteoporosis is a reduction in bone density resulting in increased brittleness, and it can affect the strength and amount of bone tissue. We all lose a slight amount of bone mass as we age, but other factors can accelerate this loss until bones are so thin they become fragile and porous. This makes them more susceptible to fractures until even a slight knock, which wouldn't even bruise a normal person, would break the limb of an osteoporosis sufferer. Women after the menopause are particularly at risk because of their dwindling reserves of oestrogen, which helps guard against it.

The US National Institute on Ageing maintains that 1 in 4 post-menopausal white women is affected by osteoporosis, and 1 in 8 men over 60. It has come to be thought of as a disease associated with ageing, but, in most cases, osteoporosis is preventable. Simple changes in lifestyle may prevent or slow down its development.

We reach our peak bone mass some time between our late twenties and forties, and then bone mass starts to be lost gradually. The best way to prevent osteoporosis after menopause is to maximize your peak bone mass by exercise, in particular jogging, weight training and biking, and by making sure you've got enough calcium in your diet, because if you don't take in enough calcium, your body borrows it from your skeleton.

Adult women should consume 1000 mg of calcium a day – the equivalent of four glasses of skimmed milk – but most of us take in less than half that amount. Eating calcium-rich foods, such as oily fish, spinach and broccoli, can guard against osteoporosis, but even that won't do a lot for you without exercise.

HRT can also guard against osteoporosis, and this is particularly necessary for young women who have had a premature menopause. If the disease has already developed, HRT cannot replace lost bone density, but it may be able to slow down or even stop further losses. Surveys have shown that women who had used HRT for 6 years or more had over a 50 per cent lower risk of fractures than women who had not.

Research is also going on into the role of vitamin K metabolism in osteoporosis. Vitamin K, like other fat-soluble vitamins, may not be so well absorbed by the elderly, and a deficiency of vitamin K may interfere with metabolism of minerals such as calcium. It's still early days and, as yet, no benefits from taking vitamin K supplements have been noted, but, in years to come, vitamin K may well prove a natural cure for osteoporosis.

Who's at Risk?

Research has shown that those most likely to develop osteoporosis are:

- women who had an early or surgical menopause
- women who have suffered with amenorrhoea (the absence of periods)
- women with a history of anorexia nervosa or those who are underweight with a small skeleton
- women who do not exercise
- women whose intake of calcium is low

- women whose mothers had the disease
- women who smoke and drink higher than recommended amounts of alcohol.

HRT

Women who have had an early menopause – that is before the age of 50 – benefit most of all from oestrogen replacement in the form of HRT because the risk of heart disease and osteoporosis is increased quite significantly if you've had a premature menopause. Dr Val Godfree, Deputy Director of the Amarant Trust (which researches into HRT and runs a menopause clinic that treats many hysterectomy and oophorectomy patients) says:

If you have a hysterectomy for endometriosis at 35, you should be given HRT until you're at least 50 and would be going through a natural menopause. Then, at 50, we'd do another assessment and perhaps a bone scan and decide whether or not to carry on with the HRT.

If the ovaries are lost, there's a case for giving pre-menopausal women extra testosterone. Testosterone and oestrogen together appear to be essential for libido, energy drive and enthusiasm. Oestrogen on its own can't replace it and testosterone on its own isn't necessary. They work together.

Dr Godfree maintains that HRT can be prescribed for virtually anyone:

If there have been problems, it's not that it doesn't suit people, it's that the clinician doesn't know enough about it. If you have a surgical menopause at 35, you've lost a lot of oestrogen and tend to need larger doses, and if women are suffering problems with HRT it's usually because of inadequate doses. With a surgical menopause the symptoms can be severe, and GPs go wrong because they are used to looking after older ladies through the menopause and they get nervy when you suggest prescribing a higher dose than the manufacturer recommends. But don't forget with younger women that lots of her contemporaries are on the Pill, which has far higher levels of oestrogen than HRT. The woman's age must be taken into account and HRT tailored to suit individual requirements. There's a lot to choose from and you need an experienced doctor to advise you.

If you're having your ovaries removed, you should talk about the pros and cons of HRT with your surgeon before you go into hospital, not have the decision sprung on you by the junior doctor the night before your operation when you're likely to be in an anxious and confused state of mind. Often surgeons put in HRT implants during a hysterectomy without any discussion whatsoever, giving the woman no choice. If there are any problems, they have to put up with them for six months, which is when the oestrogen runs out. So, get as much information as you can *before* the operation and keep your options open – don't opt for an implant.

Dr Godfree continues:

HRT can do a brilliant job in replacing your natural hormones. You don't get ups and downs like a normal cycle, because HRT gives you an average dose every day. I see ladies who'd had horrendous problems before their hysterectomies and oophorectomies, and the operation has made a wonderful difference to their life. HRT can make up for their lost ovaries as long as it's done properly.

There are very few cases where HRT is not recommended. If the hysterectomy has been done for endometrial cancer, it might not be appropriate, but it depends on the stage of the disease and each case should be judged in isolation. If it's in its early stages, it can be OK.

HYSTERECTOMY, HORMONES AND HRT

It's also not advisable if you've had breast cancer and a hysterectomy, or if you suffer from severe liver disease. But there are not many conditions, and, indeed, breast cancer patients can be given progestogen on its own and 50 per cent of them are helped by this. It has to be the woman's decision and she should be given the choice.

With HRT a lot of women have to overcome their fear of the word hormone. People associate it with the Pill, but it's very different from the Pill because what goes round in your blood naturally is the same sort of oestrogen that is in HRT. I've met a lot of very anxious ladies who don't understand what hormones are, and I try and get rid of the fear factor. Oestrogen is a collective term and there are different types of oestrogen – man-made oestrogen, oestrogen found in your body, in plants like ginseng ... it's not one substance, and when women understand that, it usually makes them feel a lot better.

Opinion is split, however, about the long-term use of HRT. There is a growing belief that the risk of breast cancer increases if HRT is taken for longer than 15 years, but only if it is taken after the age of 50. Women of 35 on HRT have the same risk of developing breast cancer as women of the same age who are *not* on HRT. But, the fact is there is still a great deal that doctors don't know about the long-term risks of HRT, and if you are over 50 you should talk to a specialist before deciding to take it, so that you are clear about its advantages and disadvantages.

Talk to your GP or your consultant before your operation and find out your options. If necessary, ask to be referred to a specialist menopause clinic. The decision as to what sort of HRT you will have should be made in the out-patients clinic when the decision to have a hysterectomy has been taken. The more information you have, the more reassured you'll feel, and the more easily you'll be able to make an informed choice.

What Sort?

HRT is available in pills, patches or implants. In pill form, it comes in a blister pack, rather like the combined Pill. These are handy to take and easiest to stop if you get side-effects, but the disadvantage of oral HRT is that most of the oestrogen is broken down by the liver, so it should not be taken by anyone with liver disease.

Skin patches look like round see-through plasters the size of a ten pence piece. They're worn on the buttock and changed twice a week, providing a constant level of oestrogen. These are often better tolerated because of the sort of ocstrogen they contain, they're unobtrusive and you don't have to remember to take a pill, and some doctors prefer them because they're kinder to the liver. Some women may suffer an allergic skin reaction to patches, and they may occasionally come off while you're having a bath.

HRT implants are usually inserted by the surgeon after a total hysterectomy and if you want to keep on with them, they're replaced every six months, usually under the skin of the abdomen under local anaesthetic. They have advantages in that once they're there you can forget about them until they have to be replaced, but they can be a nuisance if they have to be removed because of side-effects. It can take two or three attempts to find the HRT that best suits you.

Side-effects

Most side-effects wear off within the first three months, and if they don't they can usually be adjusted by a change of medication. Unfortunately, some GPs know little about HRT and tend to prescribe one brand (the cheapest) for *every* woman who walks into their surgery, rather than tailoring it to fit each individual.

Breast tenderness and fluid retention are the commonest side-effects. Pains in the legs should be reported to your GP at once, especially if the pain is in one leg. Don't stop HRT abruptly, even if you're experiencing side-effects. It should be reduced slowly.

Who Can't Take It?

- Women with liver disease.
- Women who've had breast cancer or with a family history of breast cancer.
- Women whose hysterectomy was for endometrial cancer.

Alternatives

Not every woman wants to take HRT, especially those who have had their ovaries removed close to their menopause and are therefore not suffering such unbearable menopausal symptoms.

Joan recalls her experience of HRT:

When I had my hysterectomy, the surgeon put in some implants which he told me would last for six months. He then advised me to get regular supplies of oral HRT when these wore off. I wasn't too happy about it because I prefer following a natural way of life, but I duly got my prescription and started reading all the contra-indications on the pack. It said that women with blood clotting disorders are advised not to take HRT and that worried me as both my parents died from thrombosis. So I decided against it, and even though I was 50 and approaching menopausal age, I did feel bad on and off for a few months and still do on occasions. But I have a homoeopathic remedy which has helped enormously, and I had a course of acupuncture. I also try and eat a good diet and lead a healthy life, all of which, I feel, contributes to the fact that I feel good for most of the time.

Relief of Symptoms

Hot flushes can be helped by wearing natural fibres next to the skin and avoiding nylon sheets. Don't smoke or drink alcohol or coffee late at night as these affect the blood vessels, and avoid spicy foods.

Taking evening primrose oil can help. Your doctor can prescribe drugs such as Clonidine, the Pill or beta-blockers, but all these have side-effects that are, in many cases, worse than the hot flushes.

Vaginal dryness can be helped by using KY Jelly just before intercourse or a vaginal cream called Replens. The latter is a non-hormonal moisturizer that feels similar to natural vaginal secretions and is good for overall vaginal, as well as sexual, comfort.

Some women I spoke to found acupuncture worked well at relieving menopausal symptoms. Acupuncture can stimulate your body's natural hormone production and help psychological symptoms such as anxiety, depression and irritability (see pages 31–3). It can also alleviate symptoms such as hot flushes and back pain, and can help sagging breasts and poor skin by improving muscle tone.

Aromatherapy – the therapeutic use of essential oils in body massage or (less effectively) in baths – can be useful for psychological symptoms as, properly carried out, it can relax the mind and relieve feelings of depression, memory loss and irritability. It has been shown to affect the body's hormone-producing glands.

A skilled aromatherapist can prepare a special blend of oils to ease hot flushes and back pain and to balance the hormones. The neat oil must be diluted before use with cold-pressed olive or almond oil in a concentration of 1 to 3 per cent essential oil to base (the vegetable oil), and a whole body massage will probably need about 25 ml (1 fl oz) vegetable oil and 8 to 12 drops of essential oil (or 10 drops of essential oil in a bath).

There are many oils that are suitable for the relief of menopausal symptoms, including rose oil, which is calming for psychological problems; geranium oil mixed with ylang-ylang, which, rubbed into breasts, can improve muscle tone; and tea tree oil, which can help vaginal dryness. You can administer the oils by gently massaging them in yourself or, better still, ask your partner to do it. But, use essential oils with care and, ideally get a blend prepared by a qualified aromatherapist to suit your individual requirements as some can be toxic.

Homoeopathic remedies that can help menopausal symptoms can be bought over the counter in chemists or healthfood shops, but the most effective remedies are those prescribed by a qualified homoeopath and especially tailored to suit you after a careful and detailed discussion of your symptoms. There are many available remedies, including lachesis, sepia, pulsatilla (for mood changes), belladonna (for hot flushes), graphites (for loss of libido, emotionalism and obesity during menopause), cimifuga (for depression, irritability, restlessness), caulophyllum (for nervous tension, anxiety, emotional instability, joint pains) and arnica (for backache, tiredness, aching muscles). Arnica is also available in ointment form, which is useful for post-operative bruising.

Chapter 9
GRIEF AND LOSS

A hysterectomy is more than just an operation to remove a troublesome and unnecessary organ. It involves the loss of what most of us see as the essence of our femininity and takes away our ability to bear children. Because a uterus is not necessary for life, it is often dismissed as being of no consequence by doctors after it has outlived its usefulness in terms of being able to support a pregnancy. But, although it may not be essential, its removal can have an effect on a woman's quality of life.

Many women I spoke to felt that the emotional implications of the operation are often overlooked by doctors, who concentrate on restoring them to a state of physical well-being, but pay scant attention to their state of mind. A woman may very well feel better physically after a hysterectomy, but she may also feel emotionally stressed or depressed for a while afterwards and these feelings can be confusing and worrying if they're unexpected.

Sarah suggests:

I think it would have helped if I'd talked to a hysterectomy counsellor beforehand, or been in touch with a support group. At least I would have been reassured that what I felt was absolutely normal.

GRIEF AND LOSS

As it was, I felt as though I was cracking up in the weeks after I was discharged from hospital and I couldn't understand what was the matter. I didn't know there were hysterectomy counsellors or support groups. My doctor was old school – he believed in pulling yourself together and getting on with it. That made me feel worse.

If you've ever had major surgery, you'll know what a tremendous strain it can put on both mind and body. A major study carried out in 1960 showed that a number of patients with no previous history of mental illness can suffer from severe depression after surgery, and that a hysterectomy is twice as likely to leave you with emotional after-effects than other operations.

Even taking into account that the time spent in hospital has shortened dramatically in the 30-odd years since that research was carried out, and that anaesthetics and surgical procedures nowadays have far fewer physical side-effects, the fact remains that surgery can have a traumatic effect on you mentally and physically – and the uterus carries a significance that can make its loss more poignant.

Not only is the uterus closely identified with the female role, it also plays a part in sexual response, which is often overlooked or denied (see Chapter 10). Furthermore, it is uniquely female: there is nothing comparable in a man. In a study carried out in Oxford in 1972, it was found that 70 per cent of hysterectomy patients suffered from depression afterwards, compared to 30 per cent of patients who did so after other operations. From this study, it was realized that post-hysterectomy syndrome was an actual condition.

Feelings of loss are common. For some women, it's the loss of identification with the female role. This is an essential part of our being, the unseen core of our femininity from which the cycle of life emanates. And, like all losses, it needs to be mourned.

It's not always understood that we respond to major changes and losses in our lives with grief. We all experience grief at some point in our lives. It's a natural response to loss and is normally only associated with the death of a loved one, but it can also be a response to many other kinds of losses, such as a relationship, a home or a job. It is also a very common response after a hysterectomy, and it helps if you can understand why.

Even though it is absolutely normal to experience grief after a hysterectomy, when it happens you can feel very isolated. Some women said they believed at the time that they were the only ones to have felt this way, and felt foolish or guilty for feeling so sad. This sense of isolation could be partly due to the fact that most of us have a tendency to keep grief locked away and not talk about the confusing and disturbing feelings it brings. But, it may also be that some women aren't even aware that they're going through a process of grieving. This was how Alison felt:

It wasn't until I got talking to someone else who'd had a hysterectomy and she told me how she felt this overwhelming sadness and depression for about six months afterwards that I realized it wasn't just me, this could happen to others, too. I'd been feeling guilty because I couldn't seem to pull myself together, and I'd try and snap out of it by putting on a happy face for the sake of my partner, little knowing that was the worst thing I could have done. I managed to find a post-hysterectomy counsellor and that made a lot of difference – just being helped to acknowledge these feelings, and to realize that what I felt was absolutely normal.

It doesn't help, either, when some doctors don't understand why you may feel low after your hysterectomy, because, from where they're standing, you *should* be feeling better. Even well-meaning and supportive friends and family may be puzzled as to why you're still feeling depressed weeks after your operation when you're clearly perfectly fit and recovering well, and the sympathy they gave you in those early days may well evaporate. What often happens then is that you try to suppress your feelings, even

GRIEF AND LOSS

though you may feel like screaming inside, but you only succeed in making things worse. Suppressed grief doesn't usually go away.

Grief can be expressed in a whole range of ways. Its effects can be felt in the mind and the body and the depth of grief will depend on a variety of factors. No two people will grieve in the same way – it depends on our personality and how easily we can express ourselves, and also the depth of feeling we have – a young, childless woman who has had a hysterectomy because of cancer is likely to feel the loss far more profoundly than would an older, post-menopausal woman who has completed her family. But it's impossible to generalize and some women who appear to be very positive about the operation can be hit very badly by the grieving process. Then again, some women sail through it all entirely untouched by any of it. There is a general pattern, though, and it may help if you know what it is so that if it happens to you, you can understand that what you are going through is very normal.

The initial response to loss may involve shock and disbelief, even if you were prepared for and expecting it. You may find it odd that the world is going on around you in much the same way, while inside you feel numb with grief.

This can be followed by denial, which is a defence against accepting the notion that you no longer have a womb or can bear a child. When you finally accept it, you may turn off completely and become zombie-like. Anger can play a big part in the grief process, and this is a tricky emotion to handle because most people find it unacceptable, but it can play a vital part in helping us face up to the reality of the loss. You may also feel guilt and depression and these too can be very draining. They both contain elements of hopelessness and helplessness and, as with some kinds of anger, we often turn them inwards and we can feel as though there is no future.

Alison recalls:

HYSTERECTOMY

I felt so guilty after my hysterectomy. I'm a Catholic, and my faith is important to me. I saw my womb as something special, a place to nurture and bring forth children, even though I'm 39 and I didn't want any more children. I agreed to a hysterectomy because I had the most enormous fibroid which was causing me a lot of pain, and I was having such heavy periods it started to get me down. I was anaemic and I got to the stage when I thought, I'll do anything to stop this. It's only an operation, why should it matter? I was unprepared for the guilt and grief and depression that followed. Guilt that I'd somehow indulged in a covert form of contraception, that I'd gone against God's natural way of things. Depression that an essential part of my femininity was gone. And a terrible grief that seemed to come from way down inside me. I couldn't understand why I felt like this, couldn't understand what was going on. Once the counsellor helped me to understand I was grieving for what I'd lost, it was easier to bear.

One counsellor who has helped many women who have had a hysterectomy is left with the following impressions of their experiences:

The extent of the grief that can follow a hysterectomy has different implications. There's not only a loss of a body part and the changes that implies, but also the loss of an opportunity to bear children. It's not just the operation, but the knock-on effects: a lot of women see it as a loss of womanhood and you need to think that through and accept that you can be a whole person and not have babies.

I once counselled a woman whose first child had been born mentally handicapped. Because of this she and her husband had decided to postpone having a second child, and they were just coming round to the idea that they'd try for another when she was diagnosed as having cancer and had to have an immediate hysterectomy. This was a tremendous loss for her. She was angry with the child she had even though she loved her, because that child had,

GRIEF AND LOSS

in a sense, robbed her of the opportunity to have another. She mourned the fact that she could have no more. I could help by letting her talk through it, by listening and helping her understand that it's OK to feel like that – if you like, to give her permission to feel like that.

People need to be given the space to talk about how they feel and not feel bad about it – it's easy enough to say, but it can take ages and ages of counselling. I met a woman recently who'd had a hysterectomy some time ago, and she'd not realized how scarred she would be afterwards. She'd had such an enlarged womb they'd had to cut her vertically, and the operation had left a noticeable scar all down her abdomen. She'd cried for several days afterwards and every time she looked at her body she hated it, it made her feel a sight and she didn't want her husband to see her. Although this had happened some years ago, she still felt it strongly because she'd never talked about those feelings before.

In my experience, people who go to hospital for a hysterectomy – and, indeed, any other operation – are given wonderful medical care and support, but there rarely seems to be any psychological support. Most women I've counselled don't know about support and feel they're making a fuss about nothing if they own up to feeling sad and grieving, and that they ought to just get on with it.

Working through grief can take a long time and much depends on the implications. Some people can't face up to it for a while. If they can't work through it themselves there are often other aspects, like the woman with the handicapped child who has to cope with the grief of having a handicapped child, the loss of potential for having any more children, the loss of hopes and aspirations of family life, and the shock of having cancer as well.

Once people can understand their feelings – and this can be difficult after a hysterectomy when they've just been pronounced physically fit by a doctor – they can come to terms with what's happened and move on. It's a combination of intellectual understanding and emotional understanding. That's what you're looking for.

HYSTERECTOMY

Some people try to suppress their grief because they naturally fear the hurt and pain and sense of hopelessness that grief can bring. Maybe they think it's a sign of weakness to show their emotions, but the more you *express* your grief, the quicker it will go away. You cannot hide from grief or try to lock it away, and, although it may be a painful and unwelcome experience, it is a normal and necessary one and, in the long run, it can be healing.

Not every woman feels a sense of loss or depression after a hysterectomy, but if you're aware that it *could* happen and it's absolutely normal if it does, it'll help you get through it more easily if it happens to you. It also helps to share your experiences with others in a hysterectomy support group. You should find it easier to talk about the way you feel when you're with those who've been through the same problems, and the more you can talk about your feelings and anxieties and worries, the easier it is to cope with them. If the feelings persist and don't seem to be getting better, ask your doctor to refer you to a counsellor.

Chapter 10
SEX AFTER HYSTERECTOMY

There are two myths that persist about hysterectomy. One is that once women are free from the troublesome symptoms that led them to have the operation in the first place, their sexual performances take on a new lease of life. The other is that hysterectomy can cause women to lose their desire for sex altogether. Although most doctors seem to believe that sex will be the *same* after a hysterectomy, the truth is that nobody can say for sure how the operation will affect a woman's sexual responses, because we're all different. A lot depends on how old you are when you have your hysterectomy, whether or not you've had your ovaries removed and how much importance you placed on sex before the operation.

Your doctor will probably tell you to avoid making love for between four and six weeks after your operation because it's important that the vagina has healed completely before you have penetrative sex, but clitoral masturbation or oral sex should be fine. Having an orgasm, in fact, should be good for you because it exercises the muscles and stimulates circulation. It's OK to use a vibrator, providing you don't put it into your vagina.

Many women do find their sex life improves after a hysterectomy, because they no longer have to put up with the sometimes crippling and debilitating symptoms that drove them to have a hysterectomy in the first place. Menstrual problems don't usually go hand-in-hand with a good sex life.

Jacqui's experiences of sex before and after her hysterectomy were quite different:

> *Before my hysterectomy, our sex life was virtually non-existent, because I was having really heavy periods that were lasting up to a fortnight. When I wasn't bleeding I was so exhausted sex was the last thing on my mind. I've felt like a new person since my hysterectomy, and it's certainly given my sex life a new lease of life. It was the best thing that ever happened to me.*

Not everyone is so lucky. In Chapter 9 we saw how grief can cause emotional after-effects, and this can affect your libido. But, although it was once thought only psychological factors accounted for lack of sexual desire after hysterectomy, now doctors are not so sure. Sexual response depends on both emotional *and* physical factors, and if a woman does suffer from sexual problems after hysterectomy, it can be hard to judge whether it is due to the physical changes that have taken place or whether it is an emotional reaction to the loss of her uterus or a combination of both.

The grief that can follow that loss can also exaggerate the physical changes, but this normally resolves itself after the mourning process is over. Some doctors believe hormonal factors could be at work. Researchers found that up to 46 per cent of women had difficulty becoming aroused and reaching orgasm after this surgery. Part of the reason could be that the uterus plays an important part in sexual response.

The Female Orgasm

The first stage of the female orgasm is the excitement phase, when blood pressure rises, heartbeat and breathing quicken, breasts swell, nipples become erect and muscles tense. During this phase, increased blood flow causes a woman's genitals to swell and lubricate. If stimulation continues, the next stage is the plateau phase, during which the arousal intensifies and the uterus expands to twice its normal size, so increasing sexual tension. The outer vagina swells and narrows and the inner vagina balloons up, lifting the uterus and cervix away from the end of the vagina.

The next stage is the orgasm itself. When a woman has an orgasm, her vagina and uterus contract rhythmically; the uterus contracts with the other pelvic tissues, forcing the blood out of the pelvis and genitals and back into the abdomen. The strength of the muscular contractions throughout the pelvis seem to determine the physical strength of the orgasm, and if the uterus is missing, the vagina will not balloon out in the same way. There is less pelvic tissue to fill with blood, which may result in a lessened sensation of arousal and less intense orgasms.

It has become fashionable to remove a woman's cervix along with her uterus, even if it is completely healthy, whatever her age. The reasoning behind this is that it removes a potential cancer site, but research has started to emerge which suggests that the cervix is not just another unnecessary organ and it can play a part in arousal and sexual desire. Some surgeons are now opting to leave the cervix in place for this reason.

If you've had an abdominal hysterectomy and your cervix hasn't been removed, your vagina will still feel the same. If your cervix has been removed, there will be a line of stitches there instead, and, provided the cervix was carefully taken away (see page 48), the vagina should not be any shorter. When a woman is aroused, her vagina expands and lengthens, so, unless your partner has an unusually long penis, he will not have felt your cervix during intercourse, so he shouldn't notice any difference after your hysterectomy. If radical surgery has been performed because of cancer, part of it may have been removed, making it slightly shorter.

Scar tissue can sometimes make for uncomfortable sex after a hysterectomy, depending on where the surgeon stitches. Much depends on the surgeon's skill. One woman in her seventies I spoke to had been stitched so tightly that sex was out of the question as it was far too uncomfortable: 'I expect he thought at my age I was no longer interested', she said sadly.

If you achieved orgasm before your operation as a result of clitoral stimulation, you shouldn't notice any difference in your sexual responses because your clitoris will be intact and just as sensitive after a hysterectomy. For those lucky enough to have located it, the G-spot also remains the same.

Some women reach orgasm as a result of the thrusting of the penis against the cervix and uterus, which is no longer possible after a hysterectomy, although some have found thrusting against the bottom of the vagina can partly compensate. The vaginal contractions that occur during orgasm remain the same, though. You may have to change the way you make love afterwards. Talk to your partner, and experiment with more clitoral stimulation, finger foreplay and vaginal stroking.

Sexual response starts in the head. In order to become sexually aroused, as well as finding your partner attractive, you need to feel relaxed, unstressed and free from anxiety. Most women – and indeed, their partners – are nervous about the first time they make love after a hysterectomy. They fear it'll hurt or that their sexual desire will have diminished or that they'll split the stitches and do themselves an injury. Some men are afraid of hurting their partner and it's reassuring if you've both talked through your fears with your surgeon or hysterectomy counsellor or others in a support group. Worry and anxiety are a great turn off. If you're anxious and tense, you won't feel like making love, and, if you try to make love when you don't feel like it, it'll be an uncomfortable and negative experience. Alison found this out:

> *The first time we made love afterwards, he was nervous of hurting me and I was worried it would feel different. I kept imagining this huge space inside me where my womb had been and I couldn't get that out of my head. It was a bit of a disaster, and it rather put me off for a while. But it got better - although it was a couple of months before I managed to forget about it, relax and enjoy it.*

If your ovaries have been removed and you are pre-menopausal, you will have a surgical menopause. One of the many unwelcome symptoms of this can be a loss of sexual desire, because the supplies of sex hormones – oestrogen and testosterone – have been cut off and, together, these play a part in our sex drive. The adrenal glands do partly compensate for the loss of ovarian hormones by producing similar ones, and some oestrogen is also produced in body fat, but this is not enough for a pre-menopausal woman.

Nora Coffey founded Hysterectomy Educational Resources (HER) in the USA after her ovaries were removed against her wishes during her hysterectomy and she suffered a loss of libido as a result of the surgical menopause she underwent. HER collects information on alternatives to hysterectomy and the problems the operation can entail, and Coffey claims that it's not unusual for a woman to lose her libido, as she did, after ovarian removal, and her claims are backed up not only by the many calls she has received, but also by recent research.

HRT prescribed by a skilled and experience practitioner should alleviate menopausal symptoms, including the lack of sexual desire that can sometimes follow a surgical menopause. Psychological factors associated with the menopause can also contribute to this problem, and some women have an emotional reaction to the loss of their uterus and their ability to bear children that causes them to see sex as pointless or unnecessary. A counsellor or support group can help.

Surgery can have a psychological impact that can take some time to get over. You might also have an emotional reaction to your illness as well: if your hysterectomy was performed for something very serious like cancer, the chances are you'll feel anxious and even depressed after the surgery, because the illness may not have yet been resolved and more treatment may be necessary. Some women feel that losing what they regard as the core of their femininity makes them less desirable, and this diminishes their interest in sex. Usually these feelings disappear in time, but occasionally therapy might be needed.

It's not all bad news, however: some women find their sexual desire increases after their hysterectomy. This is particularly so if they've had the hysterectomy because of a long-term debilitating problem, such as heavy bleeding, that, in the past, has rendered sex an impossibility, as Jo found:

I can't tell you what it was like to enjoy sex free of pain for the first time for years. I'd lived with endometriosis for so long and it made sex painful at worst, uncomfortable at best. It got so I'd grit my teeth every couple of weeks and think, can't put it off any longer, and my husband could sense my reluctance and it caused a lot of pressure. Since my hysterectomy, we've had a wonderful sex life – we can really relax and enjoy it. It's fantastic.

If you enjoyed a good sex life before your hysterectomy, you probably realized that the more you made love, the more enjoyable it became, the better you got at it and the more you wanted it. Sexual activity seems to stimulate oestrogen production and increase vaginal tone and lubrication, and pelvic floor exercises can help as well, so making love as often as possible after the operation is still the best way to get better at it and enjoy it more.

There is no doubt that keeping sexually active is good for you. Apart from keeping you and your partner close, you are liable to feel depressed and tense if you stop functioning sexually. Psychologist Wilhelm Reich in a study in 1945 argued that an orgasm was such an essential component in our psychological well-being that he recommended a daily occurrence for our health's sake! Like most other parts of your body, your sexual functioning can atrophy and eventually fall into disuse if you don't make use of it.

Chapter 11

A LAST WORD

If you've read this book, the chances are that a hysterectomy has been recommended to you as the best way of dealing with your problem. Perhaps you're still agonizing about whether or not you should go ahead with it. Unless you are suffering from cancer and a hysterectomy is essential, don't be rushed into making a decision. It's your body and it's up to you what happens to it.

Having a hysterectomy can be a positive and liberating experience, from a practical and emotional point of view. No more periods or contraception to worry about, freedom from the problems that led you to have the operation in the first place. A lot of women maintain that after their hysterectomy their quality of life improved to such an extent that they felt more confident, assured and happier than they'd done for years.

But it is not just any operation. It involves the loss of a very special part of your body, and it's impossible to predict what effect a hysterectomy might have on any one person. Just as every woman is unique, so her experience of hysterectomy will be, too. So, the decision to have one needs to be thought out carefully.

Whatever decision you make, I hope this book has made it easier for you. The more informed you are, the more confident

A LAST WORD

and in control you'll be – and the more likely you are to make the decision that is right for you.

SELECT BIBLIOGRAPHY

Bachmann, G. A., *et al.* 'Vaginal Dryness in Menopausal Women', *Clinical Practice in Sexuality,* vol. 7, no. 9 (1990)

Brooke, E. *Herbal Therapy For Women,* Thorsons, 1992

Carpenter, A., and Johnson, G. *Why Am I Afraid to Grieve?,* Fount, 1993

Coulter, A., *et al.* 'Do British Women Undergo Too Many or Too Few Hysterectomies?', *Social Science Medicine,* vol. 27, no. 9 (1988)

Davis, P. *A Change For the Better,* Daniel, 1993

Dranov, P. 'An Unkind Cut', *American Health,* vol. 9, no. 7 (1990)

Dranov, P. 'When the Diagnosis is . . . Fibroids: New Treatments Will Prevent Hysterectomy For Millions of Women', *American Health,* vol.12, no. 7 (1993)

Fairlie, J. *Hormone Replacement Therapy,* Women's Health, 1992

Goldfarb, H., and Greif, J. *The No Hysterectomy Option,* John Wiley & Sons, 1990

Goldin, B. 'The Effect of Diet on Excretions of Estrogens in Pre- and Post-Menopausal Women', *Cancer Research,* vol. 41, no. 3771 (1981)

SELECT BIBLIOGRAPHY

Haslett, S., and Jennings, M. *Hysterectomy and Vaginal Repair*, Beaconsfield, 1992

Hollander, M. 'Study of Patients Admitted to Psychiatric Hospitals', *American Journal of Obstetrics and Gynaecology*, vol. 79, no. 498 (1960)

Hufnagel, V. *No More Hysterectomies*, Thorsons, 1990

Ingram, D. 'The Effect of Low-fat Diet on Female Sex Hormones', *Journal of the National Cancer Institute*, vol. 79, no. 1225 (1987)

Lark, S. 'Fending off Fibroids', *Vegetarian Times*, no. 193 (September 1993)

Long, Barry *Meditation – A Foundation Course*, The Barry Long Foundation, 1982

MacGregor, Dr A. *Is HRT Right For You?*, Sheldon Press, 1993

Magos, A., *et al.* 'Experience With the First 250 Endometrial Resections For Menorrhagia', *The Lancet*, vol. 337, no. 8749 (1991)

Mayes, K. *Osteoporosis*, Thorsons, 1987

McDougall, J. 'Cutting Out Needless Fibroid Surgery', *Vegetarian Times*, no. 149 (January 1990)

Nelson, J. *The Menopause*, Women's Health, 1992

Perlmutter, C. '15 Reasons to Say "No" to Hysterectomy: Or at Least Reconsider the Latest Alternatives', *Prevention*, vol. 41, no. 6 (1989)

Phillips, A., and Rakusen, J. (eds) *The New Our Bodies Ourselves*, Penguin, 1989

Podolsky, D. 'Saved From the Knife', *US News and World Report*, vol. 109, no. 20 (1990)

Richards, O. H. 'Depression After Hysterectomy', *The Lancet*, vol. 2, no. 25 (1973)

Robertson-Steel, Dr I., and Vaughan, C. *The Treatment You Deserve*, Right Way, 1994

Saffron, L., and Aranda, K. *Fibroids*, Women's Health, revised 1993

Shreeve, Dr C. *Problem Periods*, Piccadilly Press, 1994
Sloan, D. 'The Emotional and Psychosexual Aspects of Hysterectomy', *American Journal of Obstetricians and Gynaecologists* (1978)
Tisserand, M. *Aromatherapy For Women*, Thorsons, 1990
West, S., and Dranov, P. *The Hysterectomy Hoax*, Doubleday, 1994
Zussman, L., *et al.* 'Sexual Response After Hysterectomy and Oophorectomy', *American Journal of Obstetricians and Gynaecologists*, vol. 140, no. 7 (1981)

USEFUL ADDRESSES

Acupuncture

The Acupuncture Association
34 Alderney Street
London SW1V 4EU
Tel: 0171–834 1012

Acupuncture and Chinese Herbal Practitioners Association
1037B Finchley Road
London NW11 7ES
Tel: 0181–455 5508

British Medical Acupuncture Society
Newton House
Newton Lane
Whitley
Warrington WA4 4JA
Tel: 01925 730727

Council for Acupuncture
179 Gloucester Place
London NW1 6DX
Tel: 0171–724 5756

Cancer

BACUP
3 Bath Place
Rivington Street
London EC2A 3JR
(for cancer patients and their families)
Counselling service: 0171–696 9000
Information service: 0171–613 2121
Freefone line for callers outside London: 0800 181199

Complaints

Action for Victims of Medical Accidents
Bank Chambers
1 London Road
Forest Hill
London SE23 3TP
Tel: 0181–291 2793 (for advice if you believe the clinical care you received was negligent)

Hysterectomy Legal Fighting Fund
21 Stratford Grove
London SW15 1NU (if you've had your uterus or ovaries removed without your consent)

USEFUL ADDRESSES

Counselling

British Association for Counselling
1 Regent Place
Rugby
CV21 2PJ
Information line: 01788 578328

Endometriosis

Endometriosis Society
35 Belgrave Square
London SW1X 8QB
Tel: 0171-235 4137

General

Women's Health
56 Featherstone Street
London EC1Y 8RT
Tel: 0171-251 6580
(for advice and information on all aspects of women's health)

Herbalism

National Institute of Medical Herbalists
9 Palace Gate
Exeter EX1 1JA
Tel: 01392 426022

Homoeopathy

The British Homoeopathic Association
27a Devonshire Street
London W1N 1RJ
Tel: 0171–935 2163

The Faculty of Homoeopathy
2 Powis Place
London WC1N 3HT
Tel: 0171–837 2495

Hysterectomy

Hysterectomy Support Network
3 Lynne Close
Green Street Green
Orpington
Kent BR6 6BS

Menopause

The Amarant Trust
56–60 St John's Street
London EC1M 4DT
Tel: 0171–490 1644

Osteoporosis

National Osteoporosis Society
PO Box 10
Radstock
Bath BA3 3YB
Tel: 01761 471771

INDEX

abdominal hysterectomy 45, 48, 78–9, 82–5, 88
  and going home 90, 92
  and returning to work 99–100
Aconite 30C 6
acupuncture 31–3, 111, 112
acute PID 17
adenomyosis 14
adhesions 17, 48, 49, 83
admissions procedure, at hospital 72
adrenal glands 54, 125
alcohol 18, 104, 107, 112
alternative medicine *see* complementary medicine
Amarant Trust 107
amenorrhoea 106
anaemia 7
anaesthetics 75–6, 92, 94

anger 117
anorexia nervosa 106
antibiotics 27–8
antioxidants 57–8, 96
arnica 113
aromatherapy 112–13

backache 102
baths 95
bed, getting out of, in post-operative period 83
belladonna 113
bending 95
beta-blockers 112
beta-carotene 57
biking 105
bioflavinoids 13
bladder injuries 48, 49
bleeding:
  after menopause 6, 21, 22

137

after sex 21
heavy *see* menorrhagia
between periods 6
post-operative 48
vaginal 89, 97–8
blood circulation 82
blood loss, during period 7, 8
blood sample 72
the blues 87–8
bone scans 107
bones, brittle *see* osteoporosis
bowel wind 83–4
bowels:
  emptying 76, 83–4
  injuries 48, 49
  obstruction 84
breast cancer 109, 111
bruising, post-operative 113

calcium 6, 106
cancer 26
  of breast 109, 111
  of cervix ix, 20–2, 50, 55
  of endometrium 6, 9, 22–3, 50, 108, 111
  immediate surgery 56, 69, 128
  micro-invasive 20
  of ovaries ix, 13, 23–5, 50, 54
  as reason viii
  of reproductive organs ix, 20–5
CAT scan 24

catheters 79, 80
caulophyllum 113
cervical intraepithelial neoplasia (CIN) 20–2
cervix 2
  cancer ix, 20–2, 50, 55
  removal, during hysterectomy 46, 55, 123
Chamomilla 6c 6
check-up, post-operative 91, 95
chemotherapy 25
children, lifting 95
chlamydia 17
chronic PID 17
cimifuga 113
CIN 20–2
clips, removing 84–5
clitoral masturbation 121, 124
Clonidine 112
coffee 18, 112
Coffey, N. 125
combined contraceptive pill 9
complementary medicine 27–36
complete woman, not a 39
complications, after surgery 48, 89
computer-assisted tomography (CAT) scan 24
concentration loss 104
cone biopsy 21
consent form, for surgery 75
constipation 89

INDEX

consultant gynaecologist 69–70
contraceptive pill 112
  oestrogen content 11, 108
convalescence 92–4
coughing, after surgery 81
counselling 99, 118–20, 126
crowns, dental 76
cryosurgery 21
cycling 105

D & C 9, 22–3
Danazol 10, 16
decision, making viii, 37–44, 128–9
deep-vein thrombosis (DVT) 81–2
denial 117
depression 56, 104
  post-operative 87–8, 115, 117
diet:
  fat in 13, 22
  fibre in 19
  good 57–8
  and ovarian cancer 23
  slimming 56
dilatation and curettage (D & C) 9, 22–3
Dimetriose 16
disbelief 117
discharge, vaginal 80–1, 98
discharge procedures (hospital) 91

doctors 74–6
domestic life, organizing 72–3
douche, not recommended 95
drains 79, 80
dressings 84, 91
drips 79–80
driving 94–5
Duphaston 9, 15
DVT 81–2
dydrogesterone 9
dysmenorrhoea 5–6, 43

early menopause 106
eating, in post-operative period 83
ECG monitoring 78
eggs 3
electrocautery 41
emotions *see* psychological effects
endometrial ablation 41, 43
endometrial biopsy 9, 23
endometrial cancer 6, 9, 22–3, 50, 108, 111
Endometrial Laser Ablation 43
endometrial resection 9, 42–3
endometriosis 6, 14–17, 50, 107
Endometriosis Society 17
endometrium 3–4, 7, 14
enemas 76
energy, lack 104, 107

energy flow, balance/
  imbalance 28–9
enthusiasm 107
epidural anaesthetics 51, 75–6
essential fatty acids (EFAs) 97
essential oils 112–13
evening primrose oil 6, 16, 25,
  97, 112
exercise(s) 6, 19, 60–3, 85–7,
  105–6

Fallopian tubes 2, 4, 17
fat, in diet 13, 22
fibre, in diet 19
fibroids 9, 10–13, 44
fitness, before surgery 56–68
follicle stimulating hormone
  (FSH) blood test 10
forgetfulness 104
fortnight, first post-operative
  92–4
free radicals 57–8
freedom 128

G-spot 124
gammalinolenic acid (GLA)
  97
garlic 57
Gestrinone 16
Godfree, Dr V. 107–9
graphites 113
grief 114–20
guilt 117–18

haematoma 89
headaches 102
heart disease 103
heavy bleeding *see*
  menorrhagia
herbalism 35
high-fibre diet 19
holistic approach 28–9
home, going, following
  hospital stay 90–100
homoeopathy 33–4
homoeopathic remedies 6, 30,
  113
hormone replacement therapy
  (HRT) 19, 22, 25, 106,
  107–11
  following oophorectomy 16,
    53–4, 102–3, 125
  implants 54, 108, 110
  with LHRH agonist
    treatment 11
  patches/pills 110
hormones 3, 54, 101–2
  imbalance 4, 6, 29
hospital stay 1, 69–89
hot flushes 103, 112
housework, in post-operative
  period 94–5
HRT *see* hormone replacement
  therapy
hygiene 95
hypnosis 64–6
hypnotherapists 64
hypothalamus 3, 11, 101

INDEX

Hysterectomy Educational Resources 125
Hysterectomy Support Network 99
hysteroscope 9, 12
hysteroscopic surgery 41–2

immune system 16, 58, 96
incisions, surgical 48
incomplete woman, feelings 39
incontinence 104
infections, after surgery 48, 49
infertility, and fibroids 11
intramural fibroids 10–11
intrauterine devices (IUDs) 6
invasive cancer (of cervix) 20

jewellery, and hospital stay 71
jogging 105

KY Jelly 112

lachesis 113
laparoscope 12, 15, 45
laparoscopic biopsy 24
laparoscopic hysterectomy 45, 49–50, 51, 78, 82, 100
laparoscopically assisted hysterectomy 45, 49–50
laparoscopy 14–15
laparotomy 15
laser surgery 12, 15, 21, 41
lavatory, walking to 82

leaking 7
Lee, Mr Cheng 51–2
legs, keeping moving, after surgery 81–2
letter, for GP 91
LHRH agonists 11
lifestyle 29–30, 57
lifting 95
list, of things to take to hospital 70–2
liver disease, HRT not recommended 109, 110, 111
loss, feeling of 87–8, 114–20
low-fat diet 13
luteinizing hormone-releasing hormone (LHRH) 11

Magnesium phosphate 6
medical checks, prior to surgery 74
meditation 66–7
mefanamic acid 10
memory problems (forgetfulness) 104
menarche 4
menopause 4, 7, 10, 101–5
menorrhagia (heavy bleeding) viii, 5, 6–10, 26, 44
menstrual debris 23
menstrual disorders viii, 1, 5–10
mental health 56, 64–8
see also psychological effects

micro-invasive cancer 20
mineral supplements 96
mothers, inherited predispositions 107
moving about, in post-operative period 82–3
myomectomy 11–12

natural medicines 29–30
natural menopause 101–5
navel, incision in 49–50
necessity, for hysterectomy 26
Nezhat, Dr C. 15
night sweats 103
nil by mouth, reason 77
norethisterone 9
nurses 73–4

obesity 13, 22
obstruction in the bowel 84
oestrogen 3–4, 7, 22, 125
  endometriosis role 15–16
  and fibroid growth 11, 13, 29
  and menopause 102–5, 126
olive oil 57
oophorectomy 46, 53–4, 101, 107, 108, 125
operation, date for 56, 69–70
oral sex 121
orgasm 121, 123–4, 127
osteoporosis 103, 105–7
ovarian cysts 8
ovarian follicles 3, 10

ovaries 2, 3, 11
  cancer (tumours) ix, 13, 23–5, 50, 53
  hormone production role 101–2
  post-menopausal role 54
  removal 46, 53–4, 101, 107, 108, 125
overweight 13, 22, 56
ovulation 4, 7, 29

pain relief 6
  post-operative 76, 79
partial resection 42
partner, involving 41
pelvic examinations 8, 23, 24
pelvic floor exercises 19, 62–3, 85, 104, 126
pelvic inflammatory disease (PID) 6, 17–18
periods 4
  heavy *see* menorrhagia
  painful *see* dysmenorrhoea
peritonitis 17
pessary, for prolapse 19
Pfaffenheim incision 48
physiotherapy, post-operative 81
PID *see* pelvic inflammatory disease
pituitary gland 3, 10, 16
PMS 104
polyps 6
Ponstan 10

INDEX

positive thought, power of 63
post-hysterectomy syndrome 115
pre-med 77–8
pre-operation procedures 77–8
pregnancy 4
Premarin 625 102
preventative surgery ix
primary dysmenorrhoea 5–6
Primolut N 9, 15
progesterone 3–4, 7, 102
progestogens 9–10, 109
prolapse 18–19, 45
psychological effects:
  of hysterectomy 114–20
  of menopause 104, 125–6
  on menstrual cycle 5
  and sex 124–5
puberty 3
pulmonary embolism 81–2
pulsatilla 113

quality of life 128
questions, during decision-making time 40

radical hysterectomy 21, 46
radio, and hospital stay 71
Radio Frequency-induced Endometrial Ablation 43
radiotherapy 25
Rayner, I. 51
recovery time 56

recuperation period 1, 90–100
recurrent PID 17
Reich, Dr H. 50
Reich, Dr W. 127
relaxation techniques 6, 64–8
Replens 112
reproductive organs, cancer of ix, 20–5
reproductive system 2, 3–4
resectoscope 9, 42
rest 82

sanitary pads 70, 98
scar tissue, and sex 124
secondary dysmenorrhoea 6
selenium 96
selenium ACE 16
self-hypnosis 64–6
sepia 113
sex, following hysterectomy 121–7
sexual responses (libido) 38, 54, 102, 107, 121–2, 125
shaving, body hair 76
shock 117
sickness, after anaesthesia 75–6
side-effects 9–10, 16, 27–8
  of HRT 110–11
sleep, enough 18
smear tests 20–1, 54
smoking 18, 59, 104, 107, 112
speculum 8
spicy foods, avoiding 112

spinal epidurals 51, 75–6
stitches 82, 84–5, 95, 97
stockings, for post-operative period 76, 82
stomach muscle exercises 60–1, 86–7
stress 18, 29
stroke 103
sub-acute PID 17
sub-total hysterectomy 46
submucous fibroids 10–11
subserous fibroids 10–11
support groups 99, 125, 126
suppositories 76
surgeons 53
surgery:
  physical and mental effects 115, 126
  types 45–55, 74–5
surgical menopause 101–5, 106, 107–8
Sweden vii
swimming 95
symptoms, treatment 29

talcum powder 23
Taxol 25
testosterone 54, 102, 107, 125
theft, in hospital 71
thin women, menopausal problems 105, 106
time, for making decision 39–40
tiredness 104

total hysterectomy 46
total hysterectomy with bilateral salpingo-oophorectomy 46
total laparoscopic vaginal hysterectomy 49–50
Transcervical Resection of the Endometrium (TCRA) 42–3
TV, and hospital stay 71

ultrasound scan 23, 24
unwell feeling 104
urethral injuries 48
urinary infections 89
urine samples 74
USA vii
uterus 2, 122
  abnormal growths 8
  orgasm effects 123, 124
  prolapse of 18–19, 45

vagina 2
  bleeding 89, 97–8
  discharge 80–1, 98
  dryness 102, 103–4, 112
  healing 121
  orgasm effects 123, 124, 126
  prolapse of 18
vaginal hysterectomy 45, 49, 51–2, 82
valuables, and hospital stay 71
vertical incision 48
vibrators 121

INDEX

visitors 88–9
vital force 28
vitamin A 96
vitamin B6 supplements 16
vitamin B-complex
    supplements 6, 16
vitamin C 13, 57, 96
vitamin E 57, 96
vitamin K 106
vitamin supplements 16, 18, 96

waiting list 69–70
walks 94

weight:
    gain 98, 102
    losing 19
weight training 105
Wertheim's hysterectomy 21, 46
work, returning to 99–100
wound, infection 89
wound abscess 89

yoga 6, 67–8
yogurt 58

zinc supplements 6, 16

MENOPAUSE WITHOUT MEDICINE
How to cope with 'the change'

Linda Ojeda

The menopause is just one of a number of changes that you, as a woman, will go through in the course of your life. How easily you adapt to it depends on how well prepared you are, both physically and mentally.

There are many cultural misconceptions about this phase of life. Linda Ojeda explains the real issues that lie behind the common perceptions and tells you how to treat or prevent any possible problems using natural remedies.

She also helps you to:

- analyse and improve your lifestyle
- minimize stress
- cope with hot flushes, insomnia, fatigue and osteoporosis
- develop your own personal programme of nutrition and exercise
- keep yourself healthy in mind and body.

Remember, the menopause need not be a difficult time. Armed with the information in this book, you can discover how 'the change' can be one for the better, and how it can be the start of a whole rich new chapter in your life.

HORMONE REPLACEMENT THERAPY
Making your own decision

Patsy Westcott

What can we expect of the menopause? Will it transform us from vital, energetic women into lack-lustre old crones? And how can Hormone Replacement Therapy (HRT) help? Can it fend off the misery of hot sweats, save our sex lives, and protect us against menopausal depression? Even more intriguing, will it stave off ageing and keep us young and beautiful?

Ever since it first hit the headlines back in the 1960s, HRT has attracted controversy. Few treatments have the potential to do so much good – or so much harm.

Patsy Westcott presents an objective look at the case for and against HRT, to help you take an informed decision. This book includes the latest information on:

- HRT and osteoporosis ('brittle bone disease')
- HRT and emotions
- HRT and breast cancer
- HRT and heart disease
- different types of HRT
- self help and alternative methods of treatment
- all the options open to women considering HRT today.

If you are considering HRT, this book will arm you with the facts you need to make the right choice.

NATURAL HEALING FOR WOMEN

Caring for yourself with herbs, homoeopathy and essential oils

Susan Curtis and Romy Fraser

Natural Healing for Women is written by two people with many years experience in natural medicine. It explains the different needs of our energy and repair systems and how to use the natural healing options now available. It is fully comprehensive and easy to use, and it includes:

The Repertory of Ailments: organised by the different body systems and areas of health, it covers psychological problems as well as physical ailments – from anxiety to acne and children's illnesses to cancer – and explains conventional methods of treatment and the benefits of alternative approaches.

The Materia Medica: an A to Z of alternative remedies and treatments, including homoeopathy, herbal and flower remedies and essential oils, with clear instructions on preparation and application.

Lifestyle: a unique guide to healing mind, body and spirit. It contains realistic guidelines for improving diet, exercise, sleep and relaxation techniques, complete with a cleansing programme and useful first aid kit.

For a natural approach to total well-being there is no better book.

MENOPAUSE WITHOUT MEDICINE	0 7225 2813 2	£4.99	☐
HORMONE REPLACEMENT THERAPY	0 7225 2782 9	£4.99	☐
NATURAL HEALING FOR WOMEN	0 04 440645 2	£7.99	☐

All these books are available from your local bookseller or can be ordered direct from the publishers.

To order direct just tick the titles you want and fill in the form below:

Name: _____

Address: _____

_____

_____ Postcode: _____

Send to Thorsons Mail Order, Dept 3, HarperCollinsPublishers, Westerhill Road, Bishopbriggs, Glasgow G64 2QT.
Please enclose a cheque or postal order or your authority to debit your Visa/Access account –

Credit card no: _____

Expiry date: _____

Signature: _____

– up to the value of the cover price plus:
UK & BFPO: Add £1.00 for the first book and 25p for each additional book ordered.
Overseas orders including Eire: Please add £2.95 service charge.
Books will be sent by surface mail but quotes for airmail dispatches will be given on request.

24–HOUR TELEPHONE ORDERING SERVICE FOR ACCESS/VISA CARDHOLDERS – TEL: 0141 772 2281.